やさしい医学英語
Introduction to Medical English

編集　青野淳子　前・四日市看護医療大学教授

執筆　青野淳子
　　　Daniel P Considine

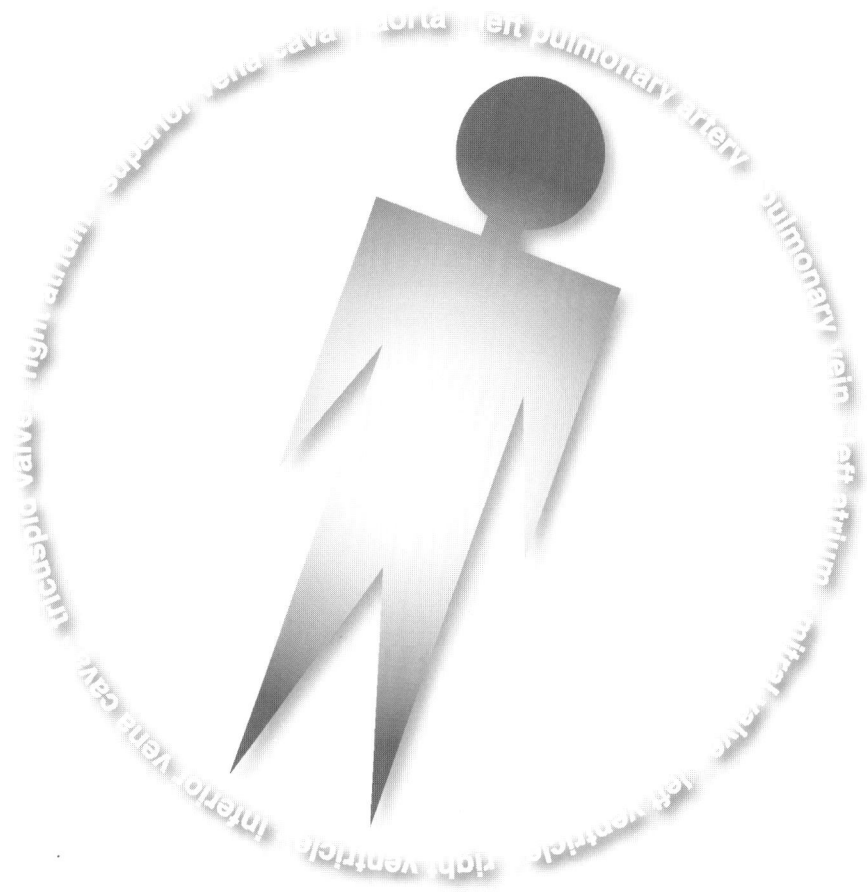

医学書院

執筆者略歴

青野淳子(あおのじゅんこ)
九州大学大学院薬学研究科博士課程修了，薬学博士
宮崎医科大学，聖マリアンナ医科大学，帝京平成大学，
四日市看護医療大学等を歴任。

Daniel P Considine(ダニエル P コンシダイン)
ニューヨーク州立大学大学院人間学研究科神経生理学修士課程，
同コミュニケーション学博士課程を修了。
米国で大学教育活動ののち来日，ライオグランデ大学日本校教授・校長を務める。
現在，法政大学等日本の大学でESL・国際コミュニケーションの教鞭を執るとともに，
医療施設および企業への英語コンサルタント，研修講師等を務めている。

やさしい医学英語
Introduction to Medical English

発　　行	2006年4月1日　第1版第1刷©
	2023年1月1日　第1版第17刷
編　　集	青野淳子
執　　筆	青野淳子
	Daniel P Considine
発行者	株式会社　医学書院
	代表取締役　金原　俊
	〒113-8719　東京都文京区本郷1-28-23
	電話　03-3817-5600(社内案内)
印刷・製本	アイワード

本書の複製権・翻訳権・上映権・譲渡権・貸与権・公衆送信権(送信可能化権を含む)は株式会社医学書院が保有します．

ISBN978-4-260-00184-7

本書を無断で複製する行為(複写，スキャン，デジタルデータ化など)は，「私的使用のための複製」など著作権法上の限られた例外を除き禁じられています．大学，病院，診療所，企業などにおいて，業務上使用する目的(診療，研究活動を含む)で上記の行為を行うことは，その使用範囲が内部的であっても，私的使用には該当せず，違法です．また私的使用に該当する場合であっても，代行業者等の第三者に依頼して上記の行為を行うことは違法となります．

JCOPY〈出版者著作権管理機構　委託出版物〉
本書の無断複製は著作権法上での例外を除き禁じられています．複製される場合は，そのつど事前に，出版者著作権管理機構(電話 03-5244-5088，FAX 03-5244-5089，info@jcopy.or.jp)の許諾を得てください．

はじめに

　これは医療分野の学生のための医学英語入門書である。医療の現場では，いわゆる横文字（略号を含む）があふれている。加えて，在日外国人も年々増加している。医療分野で仕事をするにあたっては簡単な医学英語の習得が必須の状況である。

　筆者は専門教育のかたわら約10年間医学英語の教育に携わってきた。その間，適切な教科書を求めて多くの試行錯誤を繰り返した。その結果たどり着いた1つの形が本書である。

　本書は2部構成とした。Part I では人体の構造，機能，疾病をやさしい英文で説明したのち，主な疾病の英名を中心に医学用語の学習・演習が行えるものとした。Part II では代表的な検査と処置をとりあげた。ここでは英文での説明は最小限にとどめ，患者と医療従事者との短い会話文を付加した。医療分野における英会話習得のてがかりになるようにとの願いをこめた。また検査や処置に関連する専門用語も取り上げた。

　本書の特色の1つは，各章に必要な接頭辞・接尾辞を繰り返し示したことである。これにより，対象とする学生に合わせていくつかの章のみを選択して使用することが可能である。第2に各章に略号の練習問題を付したことである。医療の現場では主に略号が使われている。略号の丸暗記は苦しいが，元の英語が理解できれば正確かつ容易に覚えられるものである。大いに活用していただきたい。第3の特色は多くの図やイラストを挿入していることである。学生にとって，わかりやすく，楽しい教科書となることを念じるばかりである。

　共著者のConsidine氏は，豊かな医療専門知識を持ち，すでに15年以上日本の大学や医療機関で英語教育や指導に携わっているベテランである。英文の大部分を彼が担当し，少量の英文と残りの部分を青野が担当した。

　本書の出版にあたって多くの専門家の援助をいただいた。石崎高志先生には医学者の立場から，杉村博子先生には英語教育者の立場から貴重なアドバイスをいただいた。またそもそも本書出版のきっかけは中島章夫先生からいただき，医学書院の七尾清様，杉之尾成一様のお力添えで出版にこぎつけることができた。支えていただいた多くの方々に心よりお礼を申し上げます。

良き年の春に，編者として

青 野 淳 子

目 次

はじめに iii

Medical Terminology（医学用語の構成）... vi

解剖学的な表示 viii

Part I The Human Body: Structures, Functions and Disorders
（人体：その構造と機能・疾病）... 1

Chapter 1　Cell, Organ and System（細胞，器官および系）..................... 2
Chapter 2　Circulatory System（循環器系）.. 6
　　　　　Disorders of the Circulatory System（循環器系の疾患）........ 10
Chapter 3　Blood（血液）... 18
　　　　　Disorders of the Blood（血液の疾患）................................... 21
Chapter 4　Respiratory System（呼吸器系）... 26
　　　　　Disorders of the Respiratory System（呼吸器系の疾患）....... 29
Chapter 5　Digestive System（消化器系）.. 36
　　　　　Disorders of the Digestive System（消化器系の疾患）......... 39
Chapter 6　Urinary System（泌尿器系）... 48
　　　　　Disorders of the Urinary System（泌尿器系の疾患）............ 51
Chapter 7　Nervous System（神経系）... 58
　　　　　Disorders of the Nervous System（神経系の疾患）............... 62
Chapter 8　Musculoskeletal System（筋骨格系）.................................. 70
　　　　　Disorders of the Musculoskeletal System（筋骨格系の疾患）.... 74
Chapter 9　Skin and Sensory System（皮膚および感覚器）.................... 82
　　　　　Disorders of the Skin and the Sensory System（皮膚および感覚器系の疾患）
　　　　　.. 87
Chapter 10　Reproductive System（生殖器系）..................................... 96
　　　　　Disorders of the Reproductive System（生殖器系の疾患）.... 100
Chapter 11　Endocrine System（内分泌系）.. 106
　　　　　Disorders of the Endocrine System（内分泌系の疾患）........ 109

Part II Examinations and Treatments（検査と処置） ……117

Chapter 12　Examinations（検査）……119
1. Blood Tests（血液検査）……120
2. Vital Signs（バイタルサイン）……122
3. Electrocardiography（ECG）（心電図検査）……124
4. Endoscopy（内視鏡検査）……126
5. Ultrasonography（超音波検査）……128
6. X-ray Examination（X線検査）……130
7. Magnetic Resonance Imaging（MRI）（磁気共鳴画像法）……132
8. Biopsy（BX）（生検）……134

Chapter 13　Treatments（処置）……137
1. Intravenous（IV）Drip Infusion（点滴静注）……138
2. Ventilator/Respirator（人工呼吸器）……140
3. Hemodialysis（血液透析）……144
4. Physical Therapy（理学療法）……150
5. Occupational Therapy（作業療法）……152
6. Dietetics/Nutrition（食事療法）……156
7. Medication（薬物療法）……158

コラム
- 医学用語の複数形 …… 5
- 病院の診療科と診察医 …… 47
- 痛みの表現 …… 57
- 数量の用語 …… 77
- 色に関する用語（連結形）…… 99

Medical Terminology（医学用語の構成）

医学用語の構成はジグソーパズルに似ている。例えば，gastrology（胃病学）は次のように3成分に分解される。

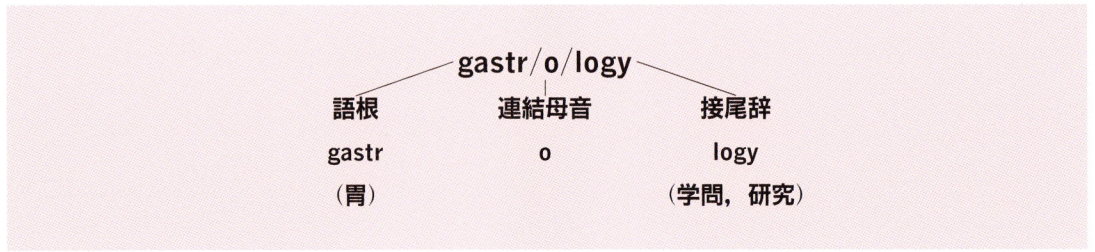

語根を hemat（血液）に換えると，hematology（血液学）となる。
接尾辞を scope（鏡）に換えると，gastroscope（胃鏡）となる。

また，接頭辞をもつ用語もある。例えば，intragastric（胃内の）は次の3成分に分解される。

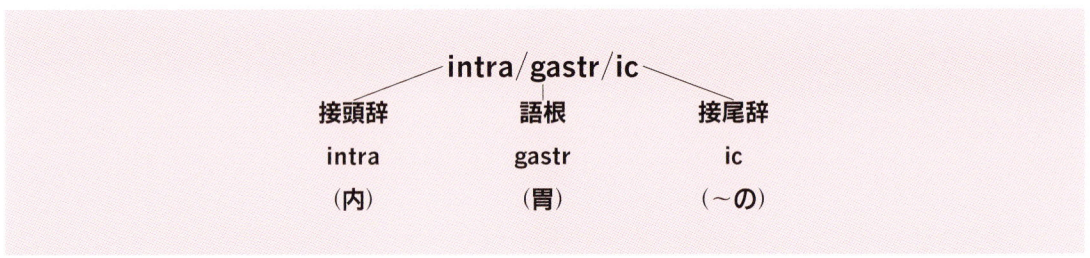

接頭辞を extra（外）に換えると，extragastric（胃外の）となる。

要約すると，医学用語の基本構造は次のとおりである。

医学用語 ＝ 接頭辞 ＋ 語根 （＋ 連結母音） ＋ 接尾辞
［連結形］

語根（root）とは，用語の核となる要素である。
連結母音（combining vowel）は，接尾辞を語根につなぐ，または語根と語根をつなぐのに使用され，それ自体は特定の意味をもたない。多くは"o"が使用される。語根に連結母音をつけたものを**連結形**（combining form）という。
接頭辞（prefix）は，語根の前にあり，語根を修飾する語である。
接尾辞（suffix）は，語根の最後につき，語根を修飾する語である。

これらの構成要素をつなぐときには次のような規則がある。

1 接尾辞を語根につなぐ，または語根と語根をつなぐときには，子音どうしの結合では発音しにくいので，連結母音(o)を加える。
　　例）gastr/o/logy　（gastrology　胃病学）

　　　　　　　　　　　gastr　＋　o　＋　logy
　　　　　　　　　　　語根　　連結母音　　接尾辞

2 接尾辞が母音で始まるときには，連結母音は省略する。
　　例）hepat/oma　（hepatoma　肝癌）

　　　　　　　　　　　hepat　＋　oma
　　　　　　　　　　　語根　　　接尾辞

3 語根と語根をつなぐときには，常に連結母音を加える。
　　例）gastr/o/enter/o/logy　（gastroenterology　胃腸学）

　　　　　　gastr　＋　o　＋　enter　＋　o　＋　logy
　　　　　　語根　　連結母音　　語根　　連結母音　　接尾辞

4 接頭辞を語根につなぐときには連結母音を使用しない。ただし，接頭辞の最後と語根の始めが母音のときには接頭辞の最後の母音を省略する。
　　例）hyp/esthesia　（hypesthesia　感覚鈍麻，触覚鈍麻）

　　　　　　　　　　　hyp(o)　＋　esthesia
　　　　　　　　　　　接頭辞　　　語根

練習問題

次の用語を構成要素に分け，用語の意味をいいなさい。
　1　neuritis　　　＿＿＿＿＿＿＿　　2　oncology　　＿＿＿＿＿＿＿
　3　electroencephalogram　＿＿＿＿＿＿＿　　4　endocarditis　＿＿＿＿＿＿＿

解剖学的な表示

Axis（軸）

vertical axis(top to bottom)	垂直軸（縦軸）
horizontal axis(side to side)	水平軸（横軸）
sagittal axis(front to back)	矢状軸（しじょうじく）（前後軸）

Direction（方向）

superior	上方
inferior	下方
cranial	頭側
caudal	尾側
anterior	前方
posterior	後方
ventral	腹側
dorsal	背側
medial	内側（身体の中心に近いこと）
lateral	外側（身体の中心に遠いこと）
proximal	近位（体幹に近いこと）
distal	遠位（体幹に遠いこと）
superficial	浅部（体表から近いこと）
deep	深部（体表から遠いこと）

Plane（断面）

frontal plane	頭面（額面，冠状面）
sagittal plane	矢状面
transverse plane	横断面

Part I The Human Body

Structures, Functions and Disorders

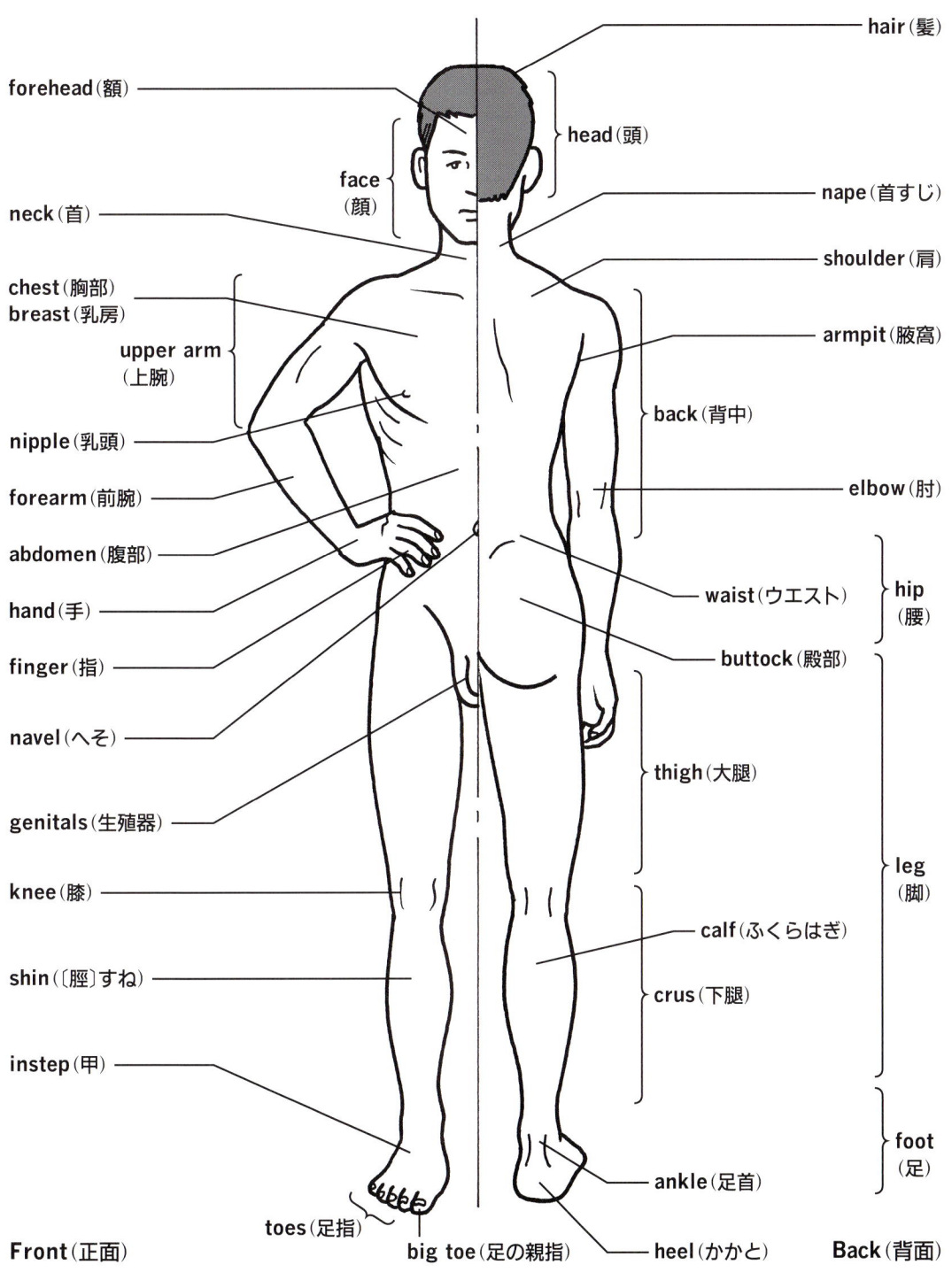

Chapter 1

Cell, Organ and System
（細胞，器官および系）

Overview

The basic part of all living things (organisms) is the cell. Some living things have only one cell, bacteria for example. More complex plants and animals have millions of different types of cells. The human body has about 60 trillion cells. These cells have different shapes (forms) and do different jobs (functions). Nerve, fat, muscle and bone cells are some of the different types of cells that humans have. A group of same type cells that work together to do a special job is called tissue. We have epithelial, muscular, connective and nervous tissues.

In the human body, several kinds of tissues work together to do a special job (function). These are called organs. The heart, lung, stomach, intestine, liver, eyes, and ears are some of the organs of the body.

A group of organs work together to perform a more complex function than any one organ can do alone. It is called a system and is the largest structural unit of the human body. The mouth, stomach, intestine and liver are different organs. They work together for digestion: the digestive system.

organism（生物体）	
bacteria (bacterium，細菌の複数形)	
trillion（1兆，10^{12}）	
function（機能）	
tissue（組織）	
epithelial（上皮の）	
muscular（筋肉の）	
connective（結合性の）	
nervous（神経の）	
organ（器官）	
heart（心臓）	
lung（肺）	
stomach（胃）	
intestine（腸）	
liver（肝臓）	
system（系）	
digestion（消化）	

Chapter 1

Most anatomists group organs of the human body into the following ten systems: skeletal, muscular, circulatory, respiratory, digestive, urinary, reproductive, endocrine, nervous, and sensory.

anatomist(解剖学者)
skeletal(骨格の)
circulatory(循環の)
respiratory(呼吸の)
urinary(泌尿器の)
reproductive(生殖の)
endocrine(内分泌の)
sensory(感覚の)

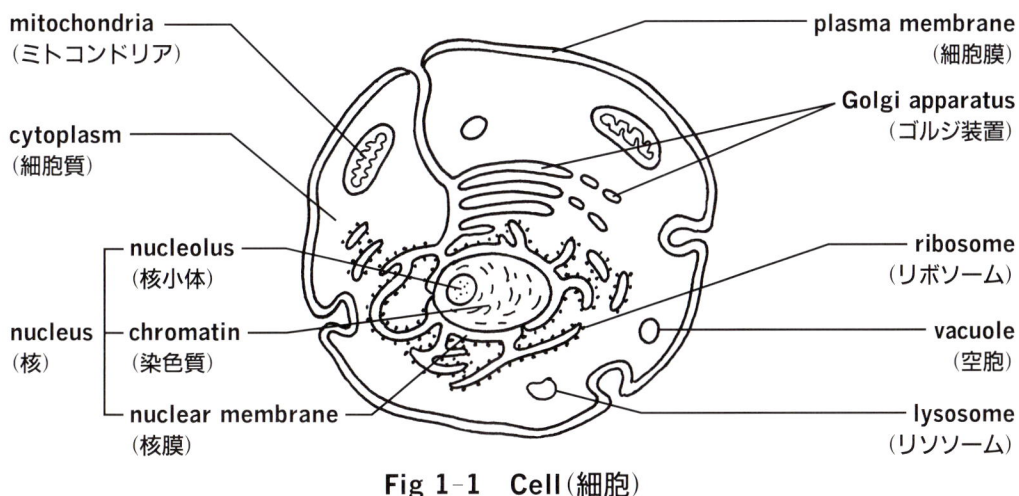

Fig 1-1　Cell(細胞)

細胞，器官および系の語根

語根の連結形	意味
cyt/o　　-cyte	細胞(cell)
hist/o	組織(tissue)

Chapter 1

Questions 1

Choose the best word from the list and fill in the blank.

1. The basic part of all living things is the _____.
2. Nerve, fat, _____ and bone cells are some of the different types of cells that humans have.
3. A group of the same type of cells that work together to do a special job, is called _____.
4. A _____ is the largest structural unit of the human body.
5. Most anatomists group organs into the following 10 systems: skeletal, muscular, circulatory, respiratory, _____, urinary, reproductive, endocrine, nervous, and sensory.

| epithelial | system | digestive | tissue | cell | muscle |

練習問題 1

1. cyto-（細胞）または -cyte（細胞）を含む次の用語の意味をいいなさい。

    1　cytolysis　_____　　2　cytotoxic　_____
    3　cytologist　_____　　4　cytology　_____
    5　osteocyte　_____　　6　chondrocyte　_____
    7　melanocyte　_____　　8　fibrocyte　_____
    9　lymphocyte　_____　　10　phagocyte　_____

2. histo-（組織）を含む次の用語の意味をいいなさい。

    1　histology　_____　　2　histologist　_____
    3　histochemistry　_____　　4　histopathology　_____
    5　histolysis　_____

医学用語の複数形

医学用語の大部分はギリシャ語またはラテン語である。それらの複数形は次のようにつくられる。

1. a で終わる単語では e を付け加える。(-a → -ae)
2. um で終わる単語では um を a に変える。(-um → -a)
3. us で終わる単語では us を i に変える。(-us → -i)
4. is で終わる単語では is を es に変える。(-is → -es)
5. on 終わる単語では on を a に変える。(-on → -a)
6. ix，ex で終わる単語では ix，ex を ices に変える。(-ix, -ex → -ices)

練習問題

例にならって表を完成しなさい。

単数形	複数形	意味
aorta	aortae	大動脈
vena cava	( )	大静脈
vertebra	( )	椎骨
atrium	atria	心房
bacterium	( )	細菌
ovum	( )	卵，卵子
alveolus	alveoli	肺胞
bronchus	( )	気管
nucleus	( )	核
centesis	centeses	穿刺
hemodialysis	( )	血液透析
peristalsis	( )	蠕動
encephalon	encephala	脳
ganglion	( )	神経節
spermatozoon	( )	精子
appendix	appendices	虫垂
calix	( )	腎杯
cortex	( )	皮質

Chapter 2

Circulatory System
(循環器系)

Overview

To circulate means to go around a circle or path. The job (function) of the circulatory system is to move blood to all parts of the body. The blood carries food (nutrients) and fresh oxygen (O_2) to the cells and carries away the waste and carbon dioxide (CO_2). We will talk about the blood in the next chapter.

The two important parts of the circulatory system are the heart and the blood vessels (tubes). The blood vessels which go out from the heart are called arteries and they carry fresh oxygen (O_2) and this makes the blood red color.* The vessels which go into the heart are called veins and they have carbon dioxide (CO_2) which makes the blood blue.**

The heart is the pump of the circulatory system, but it functions like two pumps, a right side pump and a left side pump. The right side pump of the heart receives the blood from the body through the veins and sends it to the lungs where the CO_2 is pushed out. New fresh blood with O_2 comes out of the lungs and enters the left side of the heart and is then sent out to the body through the arteries.

circulate(循環する)
circle(円，輪)
path(小路)
function(機能)
nutrient(養分)
oxygen(O_2)(酸素)
waste(老廃物)
carbon dioxide (CO_2)(二酸化炭素)
arteries (artery，動脈の複数形)
vein(静脈)
*,**肺循環(肺動脈，肺静脈)は例外
function(はたらく)
lung(肺)

Chapter 2

As we said before, the heart has two pumps, and each pump has a small top space called an atrium. The bottom space (chamber) of each pump is called the ventricle. The right atrium receives blood from the body and pushes it into the right ventricle. There is a special door called a valve, tricuspid valve, which opens only one way. This stops the blood from going back into the right atrium. The blood with the fresh oxygen leaves the lungs and goes into the left atrium. It moves through the one-way valve, mitral valve, into the left ventricle. The left ventricle pushes the blood out through the aorta to the rest of the body.

atrium (atria, 心房の複数形)
chamber (部屋)
ventricle (心室)
valve (弁)
tricuspid valve (三尖弁)
mitral valve (僧帽弁)
aorta (大動脈)

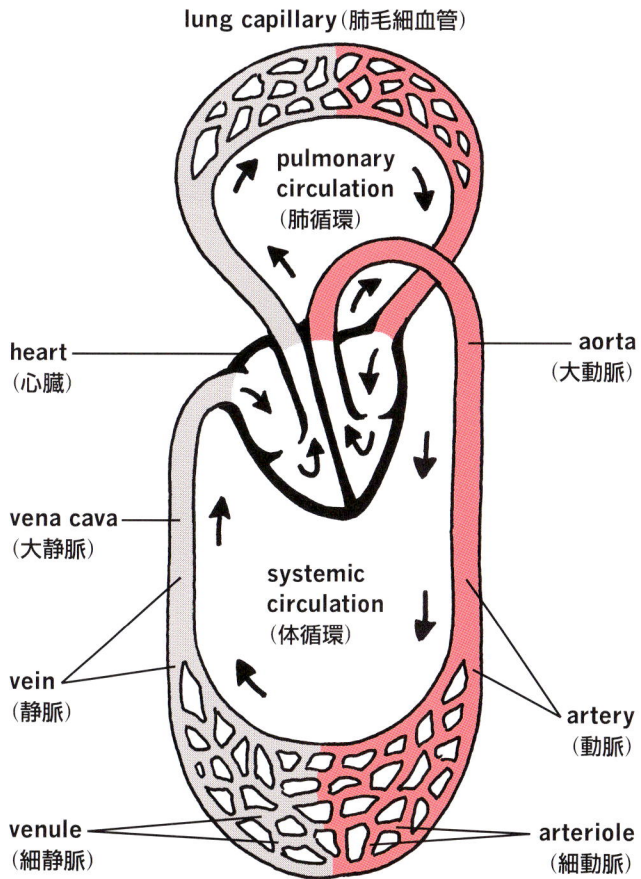

Fig 2-1   Circulation of the blood (血液の循環)

Chapter 2

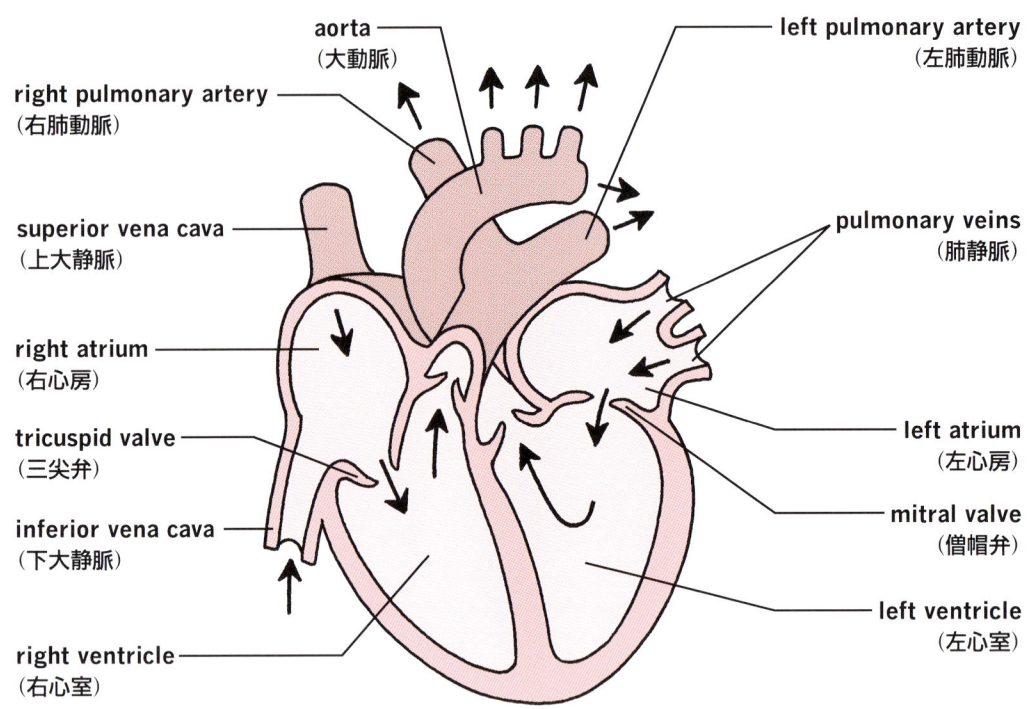

Fig 2-2 Four chambers of heart and blood flow
（心臓の 4 つの部屋と血液の流れ）

Questions 2(a)

Choose the best word from the list and fill in the blank.

1. The blood vessels which go out from the heart are called _____.
2. The blood vessels which go into the heart are called _____.
3. The top part (chamber) of the heart is called the _____ and the bottom part (chamber) of the heart is called the _____.
4. There is a special door called a _____ which opens only one way.
5. The _____ ventricle pushes the blood out through the aorta to the rest of the body.

| left | right | arteries | ventricle | valve | veins |
| atrium | venules | | | | |

Chapter 2

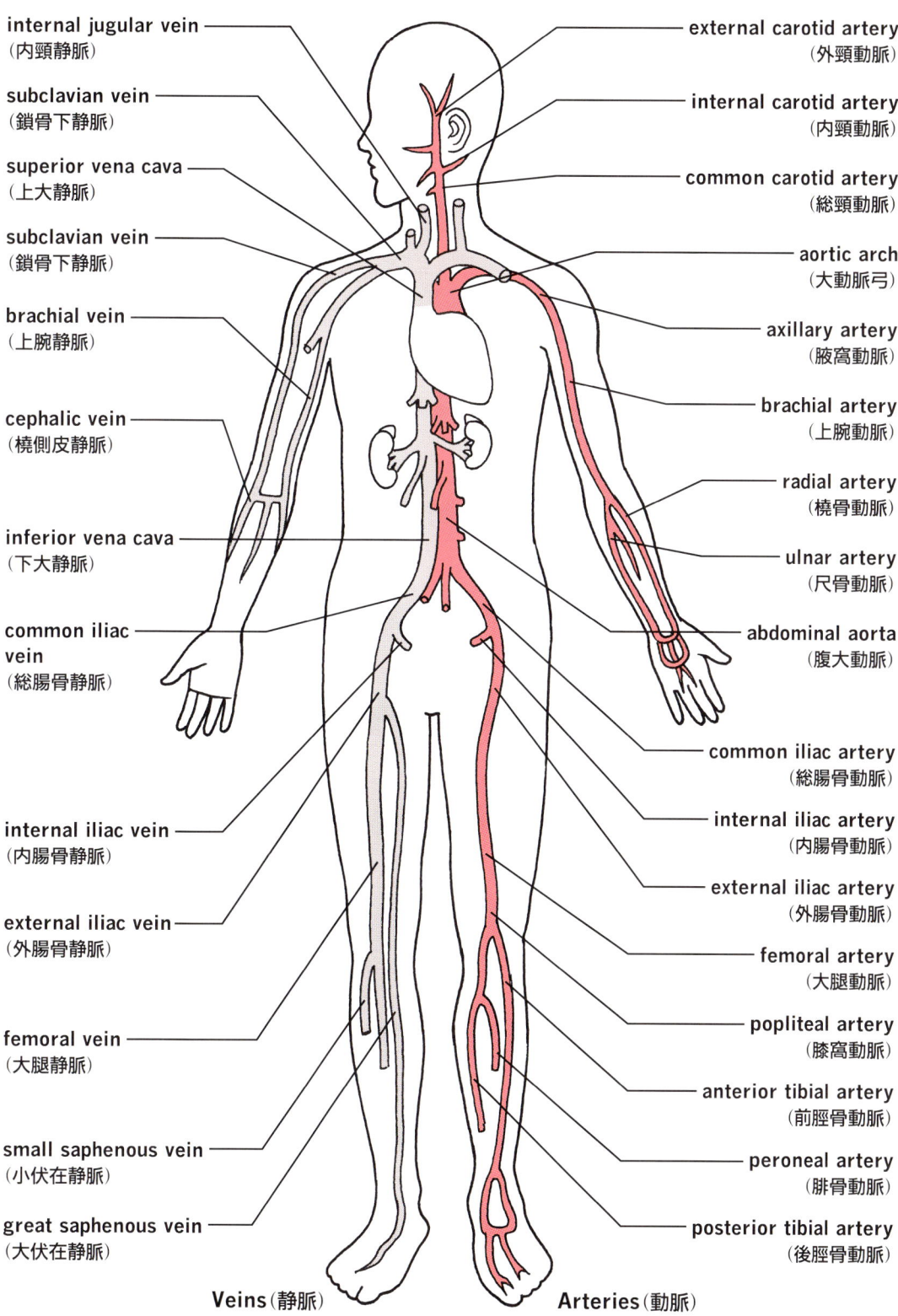

Fig 2-3 Blood vessels

Chapter 2

Disorders of the Circulatory System
（循環器系の疾患）

The arteries have walls which are pretty strong and flexible (elastic like a balloon). Cholesterol plaques are hard, thick substances that attach (connect) to the inside of the artery walls. With age these plaques make the walls hard and inflexible (not elastic). Also, these plaques grow bigger and make the inside of the wall narrow so that blood does not move through the artery very easily. This problem is called atherosclerosis and is a type of arteriosclerosis.

You can imagine that if the artery becomes very narrow then blood stops moving completely. This is called thromboembolism by blood clotting. When the blood cannot go to some part of the body those tissues will not get oxygen and will be injured or die. When we have a blood clot in an artery to the brain we get a stroke (death of brain tissue). When we have a clot in an artery to the heart muscle (coronary artery), we get a heart attack (death of heart muscle). Doctors call this a myocardial infarction or MI. The most common symptom (sign) of a heart attack is pain and pressure in the chest and the upper arm. It does not go away with rest or taking nitroglycerine.

We mentioned that there are four chambers in the heart for moving the blood around. There is a rhythm or pulse to the

---

elastic（弾力のある）

plaques（プラーク，斑）

substances（物質）

atherosclerosis
（粥状硬化症）
arteriosclerosis
（動脈硬化症）

thromboembolism
（血栓塞栓症）

clot（血塊）

stroke（発作，脳卒中）

coronary artery
（冠状動脈）

myocardial infarction
（心筋梗塞）

symptom（症状）

nitroglycerine
（ニトログリセリン）

pulse（脈拍）

heart pumping. Sometimes when we have a heart attack, lower chambers of the heart (ventricles) start to beat very fast and irregularly. This is called ventricular fibrillation. The blood does not move through the heart and, therefore, it seems to stand still. We call this cardiac arrest. Since the blood is not going to any part of the body, there can be permanent brain damage and death unless the heart can become normal within five minutes.

Angina is another pain in the heart area, but is not as bad as a heart attack. A heart attack results in permanent damage to the heart muscle. After a heart attack, the damaged portion of the heart is left with a scar. If we have many heart attacks or a heart attack with extensive muscle damage, the heart becomes very weak and develops heart failure (heart pumping declines).

ventricle(心室)
ventricular fibrillation(心室細動)
cardiac arrest(心停止)
angina(狭心症)
scar(瘢痕)
heart failure(心不全)

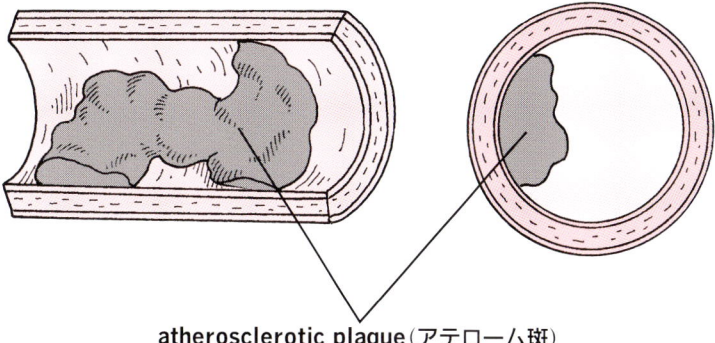

atherosclerotic plaque(アテローム斑)

Fig 2-4　Atherosclerosis(粥状硬化症)

Chapter 2

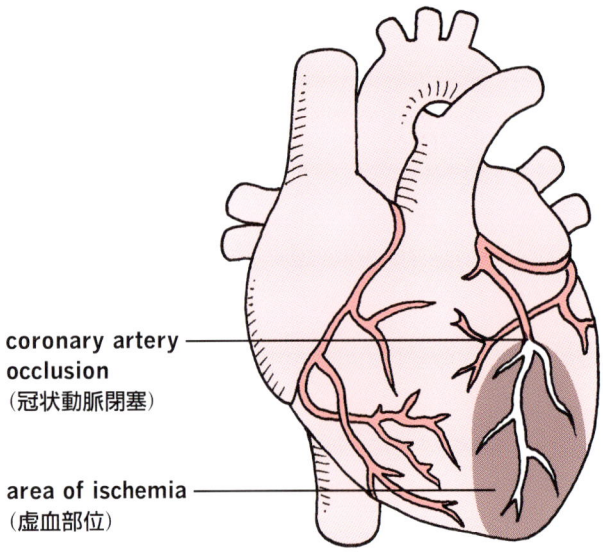

Fig 2-5　Myocardial ischemia（心筋虚血）

Questions　2(b)

Choose the best word from the list and fill in the blank.

1. Cholesterol _____ are hard, thick substances attached to the inside of the arterial walls.
2. When we have a clot in an artery to the brain, we get a _____.
3. When we have a clot in an artery to the heart muscle, we get a _____.
4. Very fast and irregular beating of ventricles is called ventricular _____.
5. _____ is another pain in the heart area, but is not as bad as a heart attack.
6. Many heart attacks may develop _____ (heart pumping declines).

| heart failure | cardiac arrest | myocardial infarction | stroke |
| arteriosclerosis | angina | fibrillation | plaques |

Chapter 2

Vocabulary

heart (cardiac) failure	心不全
acute heart failure (AHF)	急性心不全
chronic heart failure (CHF)	慢性心不全
congestive heart failure (CHF)	うっ血性心不全
ischemia	虚血
ischemic heart disease	虚血性心疾患
angina pectoris	狭心症
myocardial infarction (MI)	心筋梗塞
arrhythmia	不整脈
cardiac arrhythmia	心律動異常不整脈
sinus arrhythmia	洞性不整脈
bradycardia	徐脈
tachycardia	頻脈
flutter	粗動
fibrillation	細動
atrial fibrillation (Af)	心房細動
ventricular fibrillation (Vf)	心室細動
asystole	不全収縮
systole	心収縮
extrasystole, premature beat	期外収縮
diastole	心拡張
cardiac hypertrophy	心肥大
heart block	心臓ブロック
atrial septum defect (ASD)	心房中隔欠損症
ventricular septum defect (VSD)	心室中隔欠損症
patent ductus arteriosus	動脈管開存症
cardiogenic shock	心原性ショック
arteriosclerosis	動脈硬化症
aneurysm	動脈瘤
aortic aneurysm	大動脈瘤
varicose vein	静脈瘤
esophageal varix	食道静脈瘤
thrombus	血栓
embolus	塞栓
edema	浮腫

Chapter 2

hypertension	高血圧症
essential hypertension	本態性高血圧
secondary hypertension	二次性高血圧
hypotension	低血圧症
orthohypotension	起立性低血圧

接頭辞・接尾辞

接頭・接尾	意味	例
a-	無，不，非(not)	asystole, arrhythmia
brady-	緩徐(slow)	bradycardia
ortho-	まっすぐな(correct, proper)	orthohypotension
tachy-	急速(quick)	tachycardia
hyper-	過剰，正常範囲を超えている(above, over)	hypertrophy, hypertension
hypo-	欠乏，正常以下(under)	hypotension
-ia	〜症(異常な状態，条件)	arrhythmia, bradycardia, tachycardia
-osis	〜症(疾病の過程・状況・状態)	arteriosclerosis
-trophy	食物，栄養(nourishment)	hypertrophy

循環器系の語根

語根の連結形	意味
card/o, cardi/o	心臓(heart)
pericard/o, pericardi/o	心膜(pericardium)
valv/o	弁(valve)
angi/o, vas/o	血管(blood vessel)
aort/o	大動脈(aorta)
arter/i, arteri/o	動脈(artery)
ven/o, phleb/o	静脈(vein)
aneurysm/o	膨満(distension)
sphygm/o	脈(pulse)
thromb/o	血栓(thrombus)
ather/o	血管壁の脂肪プラーク(斑)

Chapter 2

練習問題 2

1. cardi-（心臓）を含む次の用語の意味を言いなさい。
   1. carditis _____　　2. cardiomegaly _____
   3. cardioscope _____　　4. cardiograph _____
   5. cardiogram _____　　6. tachycardia _____
   7. bradycardia _____

2. -plasty（形成術）とつないで次の用語をつくりなさい。
   1. 動脈形成術 _____　　2. 静脈形成術 _____
   3. 血管形成術 _____

3. -sclerosis（硬化症）とつないで次の用語をつくりなさい。
   1. 動脈硬化症 _____　　2. 静脈硬化症 _____

4. -graphy（造影法，記録法）とつないで次の用語をつくりなさい。
   1. 動脈造影法 _____　　2. 静脈造影法 _____
   3. 血管造影法 _____　　4. 心電図記録法 _____

5. angio-（血管）を含む次の用語の意味を言いなさい。
   1. angiogram _____　　2. angiocardiogram _____
   3. angiocarditis _____　　4. angioma _____
   5. angiocardiography _____　　6. angiocardiopathy _____

6. 次の用語の意味を言いなさい。
   1. mitral stenosis _____　　2. aortic stenosis _____
   3. mitral regurgitation _____　　4. aortic regurgitation _____
   5. pericarditis _____　　6. balloon angioplasty _____

7. 生体における血液の流れ(1〜14)について英語の名称を言いなさい。

   (1)肺静脈 → (2)左心房 → (3)左心室 → (4)大動脈 → (5)動脈 → (6)細動脈 → (7)組織毛細血管 → (8)細静脈 → (9)静脈 → (10)大静脈 → (11)右心房 → (12)右心室 → (13)肺動脈 → (14)肺 → (1)肺静脈

Chapter 2

8．日本語の意味を調べなさい。

循環器系の略語

AED	automated external defibrillator	
Af	atrial fibrillation	
AR	aortic regurgitation	
AS	aortic stenosis	
ASD	atrial septum defect	
BP	blood pressure	
CA	cardiac arrest	
CAD	coronary artery diseases	
CCU	cardiac care unit coronary care unit	
CHD	congenital heart disease	
CHF	congestive heart failure chronic heart failure	
CPR	cardiopulmonary resuscitation	
CVS	cardiovascular system	
ECG, EKG	electrocardiogram electrocardiograph	
ECMO	extracorporeal membrane oxygenator	
IABP	intra-aortic balloon pumping	
IVC	inferior vena cava	
LVAD	left ventricular assist device	
MI	myocardial infarction	
MR	mitral regurgitation	
MS	mitral stenosis	

PTCA	percutaneous transluminal coronary angioplasty	
PCPS	percutaneous cardiopulmonary support	
SVC	superior vena cava	
Vf	ventricular fibrillation	
VSD	ventricular septum defect	

Chapter 3

Blood
（血液）

Overview

Without blood, the human body would stop working. Blood lets us live every minute. It carries oxygen to the cells and carbon dioxide away from the cells. Blood lets us grow by carrying food (nutrients). And it carries hormones, from our glands, to all parts of our body. And finally, blood gives us health. It has special cells to fight disease and it carries waste and poisons to the kidneys.

Whole blood is made of plasma (55%) and blood cells (45%). We can think of blood as liquid with small things floating (suspended) inside. Plasma is the straw-colored liquid part, almost 90% water. The floating parts are the blood cells. Plasma is like the stream that carries the fish (blood cells). Plasma has (contains) nutrients, hormones, antibodies and waste materials.

There are three kinds of blood cells. Red blood cells (erythrocytes), white blood cells (leukocytes) and platelets (thrombocytes). Red blood cells have hemoglobin that carries oxygen. Their shape is like a plate (disc). New cells are made in the bone marrow and they live about 120 days. The

oxygen（酸素）
carbon dioxide（二酸化炭素）
gland（腺）
nutrients（栄養分）
waste（老廃物）
poison（毒物）

plasma（血漿）
floating（浮かんでいる）
suspended（懸濁した）
straw-colored（淡黄色の）
liquid（液体）
nutrient（栄養物質）
antibody（抗体）

erythrocyte（赤血球）
leukocyte（白血球）
platelet（血小板）
thrombocyte（血小板）
bone marrow（骨髄）

Chapter 3

old cells are destroyed by the spleen.

White blood cells are called leukocytes. *Leuko* (*leuco*) means white and *cyte* means cell. They are also called phagocytes (*phago* means to eat). There are five(5) different leukocytes and they are irregular in shape. These cells fight bacteria and disease. They can move through the walls of the blood vessels (tubes).

Platelets are the smallest of the blood cells. They are actually pieces of bone marrow cells. They help to block the blood from going out if we have a cut. This is called clotting or coagulation.

spleen（脾臓）

phagocyte（貪食細胞）

clotting（凝固）
coagulation（凝固）

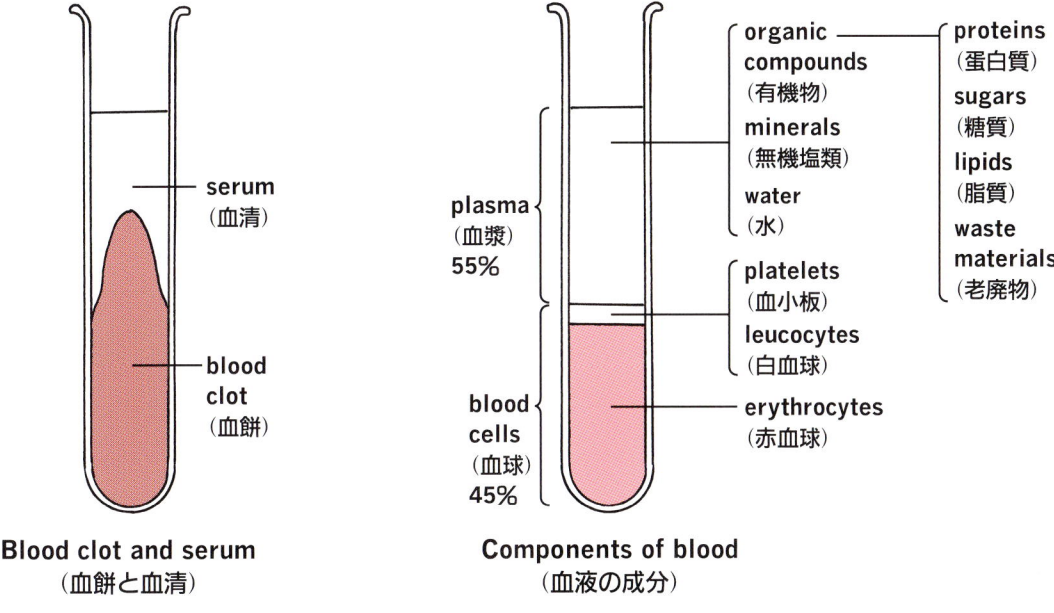

Fig 3-1 Blood

Chapter 3

Questions 3(a)

Choose the best word from the list and fill in the blank.

1. Whole blood is made of _____ and blood cells.
2. Plasma has (contains) nutrients, _____, antibodies and waste materials.
3. Red blood cells have _____ that carries oxygen.
4. New red blood cells are made in the _____.
5. The old red blood cells are destroyed by the _____.
6. White blood cells fight _____ and disease.
7. _____ help to block the blood from going out if we are cut.

platelets	bacteria	hormones	phagocytes	bone marrow
plasma	spleen	hemoglobin	coagulation	

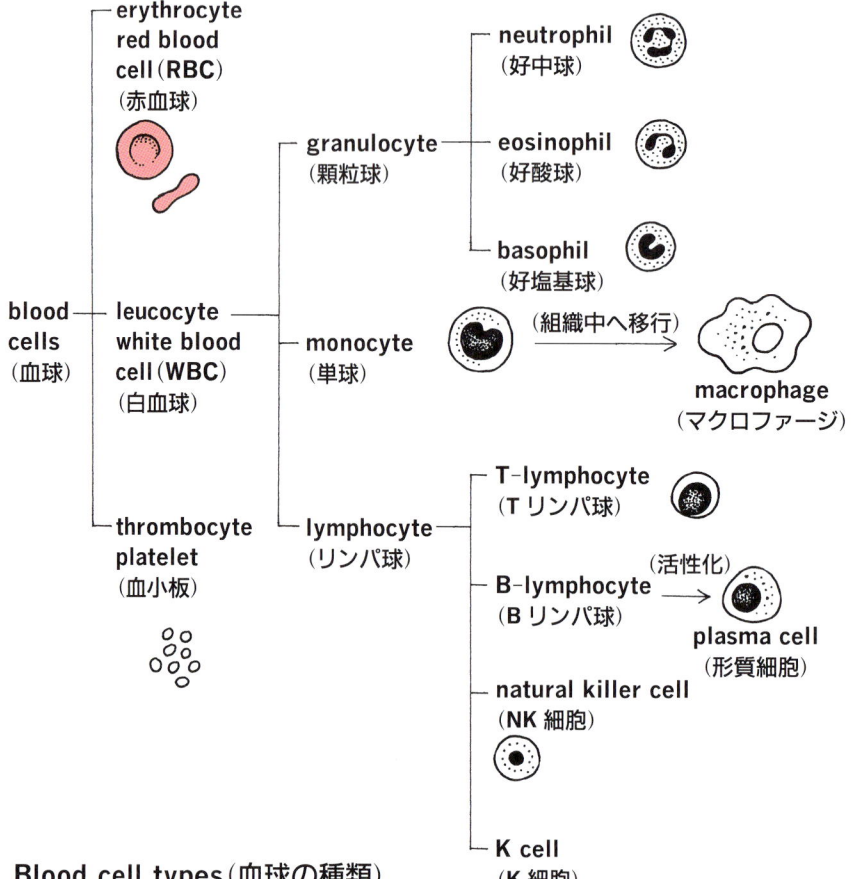

Fig 3-2 Blood cell types（血球の種類）

Chapter 3

Disorders of the Blood
（血液の疾患）

Anemia is the most well known and common blood disorder. The main problem is that not enough oxygen is going to the cells of the body. It occurs when the number of healthy red blood cells decreases in the body or they can not carry oxygen to the cells. There can be many causes for this problem.

Maybe there is not enough iron in the bone marrow. Then it cannot make enough hemoglobin and red blood cells. This is called iron-deficiency anemia and is often caused by poor nutrition.

Megaloblastic anemia may be caused by not enough vitamins. Folic acid and vitamin B_{12} are necessary to produce normal red blood cells. Aplastic anemia occurs when the bone marrow does not make some important parts of red blood cells.

Another reason for anemia is destruction of red blood cells. Hemolytic anemia occurs when red blood cells are destroyed prematurely (when they are still healthy). Sometimes, our immune system mistakes red blood cells for foreign invaders and begins destroying them. This is called autoimmune hemolytic anemia.

anemia	（貧血）
common	（普通の，よくある）
iron	（鉄）
bone marrow	（骨髄）
iron-deficiency	（鉄欠乏性）
megaloblastic	（巨赤芽球性の）
folic acid	（葉酸）
aplastic	（形成不全性の）
destruction	（破壊）
immune system	（免疫系）
foreign invaders	（外来の侵入者，異物）
autoimmune	（自己免疫性の）
hemolytic	（溶血性の）

Chapter 3

Of course the most common form of anemia is when we lose blood because of injury, surgery or a problem with the blood's clotting mechanism.　One of the major symptoms of anemia is that we feel tired (fatigue).

injury（外傷）
surgery（手術）
symptoms（症状）
fatigue（疲労）

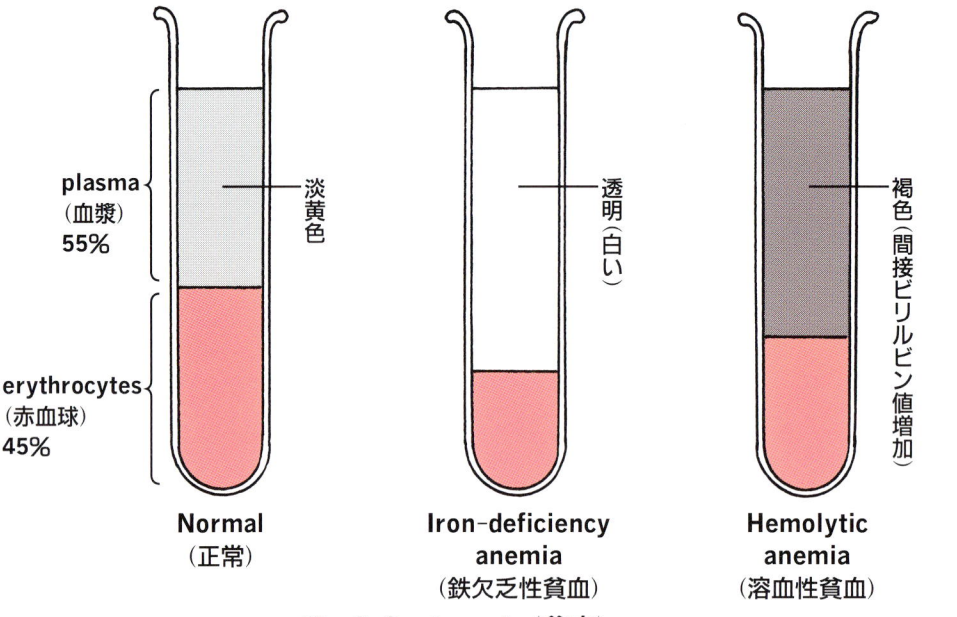

Fig 3-3　Anemia（貧血）

Questions　3(b)

Choose the best word from the list and fill in the blank.

1. The main problem of anemia is that enough _____ is not going to the cells of the body.
2. _____ is necessary to make hemoglobin and red blood cells.
3. Folic acid and _____ are necessary for production of normal red blood cells.
4. The bone marrow does not make some important parts of red blood cells in _____ anemia.
5. Sometimes our own _____ system causes anemia.
6. One of the major symptoms of anemia is that we feel _____.

aplastic	oxygen	iron-deficiency	immune	iron
fatigue	megaloblastic		vitamin B$_{12}$	

Chapter 3

Vocabulary

anemia	貧血
iron-deficiency anemia	鉄欠乏性貧血
megaloblastic anemia	巨赤芽球性貧血
hemolytic anemia	溶血性貧血
pernicious anemia	悪性貧血
aplastic anemia	再生不良性貧血
polycythemia, erythrocytosis	多血症（赤血球増加症）
thrombocytopenia	血小板減少症
disseminated intravascular coagulation (DIC)	播種性血管内凝固症候群
hemophilia	血友病
leukopenia	白血球減少症
lymphopenia	リンパ球減少症
leukemia	白血病
lymphoma	リンパ腫
splenomegaly	巨脾腫（脾臓の腫脹）

血液に関する接頭辞・接尾辞

接頭・接尾	意味	例
a-, an-	無，不，非(not)	aplastic anemia
-emia, -aemia, -hemia	～な血液を有する状態，（血液中に～を有する状態）	anemia, leukemia, polycythemia
-penia	欠乏(poverty)	leukopenia, lymphopenia
-oma	腫瘍，新生物	lymphoma
-osis	～症（疾病の過程・状況・状態）	erythrocytosis
-megaly	肥大，巨大	splenomegaly

Chapter 3

血液に関する語根

語根の連結形	意味
hem/o, hemat/o	血液(blood)
ser/o	血清(serum)
plasm/o	血漿(plasma)
erythr/o	赤色(red)
reticul/o	網状(net)
leuk/o, leuc/o	白色(white)
cyt/o	細胞(cell)
blast/o	芽細胞(embryonic cell)
lymph/o	リンパ(lymph)
myel/o	髄(marrow)
splen/o	脾臓(spleen)
thromb/o	血栓(thrombus)

練習問題3

1. -cyte（細胞）とつないで次の用語をつくりなさい。
   1　赤血球　　　＿＿＿＿＿＿＿＿　2　白血球　　　＿＿＿＿＿＿＿＿
   3　血小板　　　＿＿＿＿＿＿＿＿　4　顆粒球　　　＿＿＿＿＿＿＿＿
   5　リンパ球　　＿＿＿＿＿＿＿＿　6　血液細胞　　＿＿＿＿＿＿＿＿

2. -lysis（分解，崩壊）とつないで次の用語をつくりなさい。
   1　溶血　　　　＿＿＿＿＿＿＿＿　2　血栓崩壊　　＿＿＿＿＿＿＿＿
   3　フィブリン溶解＿＿＿＿＿＿＿＿

3. -penia（減少症）とつないで次の用語をつくりなさい。
   1　白血球減少症　＿＿＿＿＿＿＿　2　リンパ球減少症　＿＿＿＿＿＿＿

4. -oma（腫瘍）とつないで次の用語をつくりなさい。
   1　骨髄腫　　　＿＿＿＿＿＿＿＿　2　リンパ腫　　＿＿＿＿＿＿＿＿
   3　血腫　　　　＿＿＿＿＿＿＿＿　4　芽細胞腫　　＿＿＿＿＿＿＿＿

Chapter 3

5．日本語の意味を調べなさい。

血液に関する略語

BUN	blood urea nitrogen	
CBC	complete blood cell count	
DIC	disseminated intravascular coagulation	
ESR	erythrocyte sedimentation rate	
FBS	fasting blood sugar	
FDP	fibrin/fibrinogen degradation products	
Hb, Hgb	hemoglobin	
Hct	hematocrit	
HLA	human leucocyte antigen	
MCH	mean corpuscular (red cell) hemoglobin	
MCHC	mean corpuscular hemoglobin concentration	
MCV	mean corpuscular volume	
PT	prothrombin time	
RBC	red blood cell	
WBC	white blood cell	

Chapter 4

Respiratory System
（呼吸器系）

Overview

The job (function) of the respiratory system is to put oxygen (O_2) into the blood and take out carbon dioxide (CO_2). We breathe in air through the mouth and nose and it goes down a pipe called the trachea. The trachea divides into two big tubes called bronchi. One goes to the left lung and the other goes to the right lung. It looks like an upside-down Y.

Inside the lung the tubes divide into smaller and smaller tubes called bronchioles. At the end of these little tubes are very small air sacs (like very tiny balloons) called alveoli.

Very small blood vessels (pipes/tubes) called capillaries are (wrapped) around the alveoli. These capillaries have very thin walls and many of them touch each alveolus. The walls are so thin and close to each other that the air easily seeps through. In this way, oxygen seeps into the bloodstream and carbon dioxide, in the bloodstream, seeps out the alveoli. It (CO_2) is then removed from the body when we breathe out.

There is a big muscle under the lungs and above the stomach.

oxygen（酸素）
carbon dioxide（二酸化炭素，炭酸ガス）
breathe（息をする）
trachea（気管）
bronchi（気管支，bronchus の複数形）
upside-down（逆さまの）

bronchioles（細気管支）
alveoli（肺胞，alveolus の複数形）

capillaries（毛細血管，capillary の複数形）

seep（しみ出る）

Chapter 4

This muscle, called the diaphragm, moves up and down to push the air in and out of the lungs.

diaphragm（横隔膜）

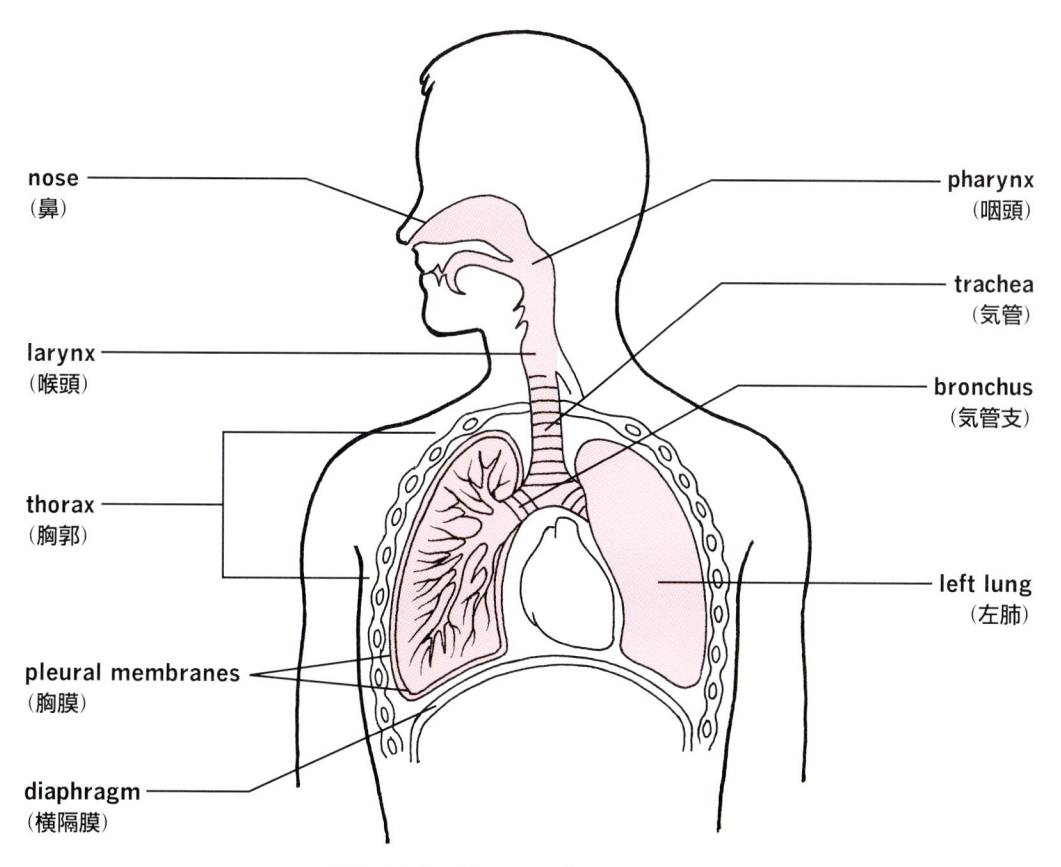

- nose（鼻）
- pharynx（咽頭）
- trachea（気管）
- larynx（喉頭）
- bronchus（気管支）
- thorax（胸郭）
- left lung（左肺）
- pleural membranes（胸膜）
- diaphragm（横隔膜）

Fig 4-1　Respiratory system

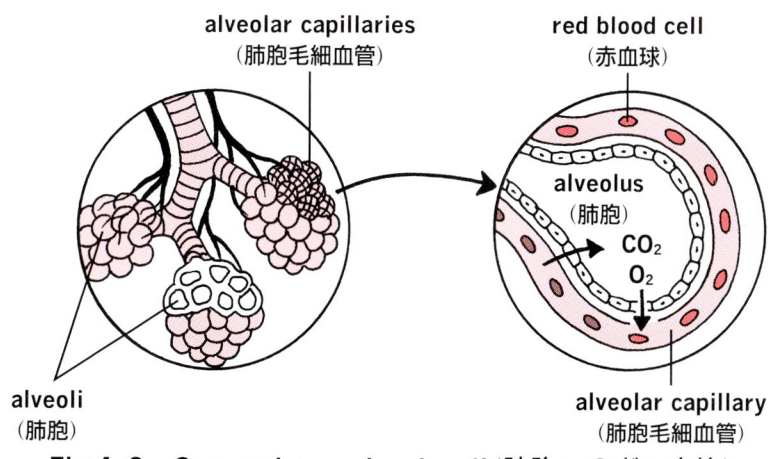

- alveolar capillaries（肺胞毛細血管）
- red blood cell（赤血球）
- alveolus（肺胞）
- CO_2
- O_2
- alveoli（肺胞）
- alveolar capillary（肺胞毛細血管）

Fig 4-2　Gas exchange in alveoli（肺胞でのガス交換）

Chapter 4

diaphragm in
inspiration
（吸息時の横隔膜）

diaphragm in
expiration
（呼息時の横隔膜）

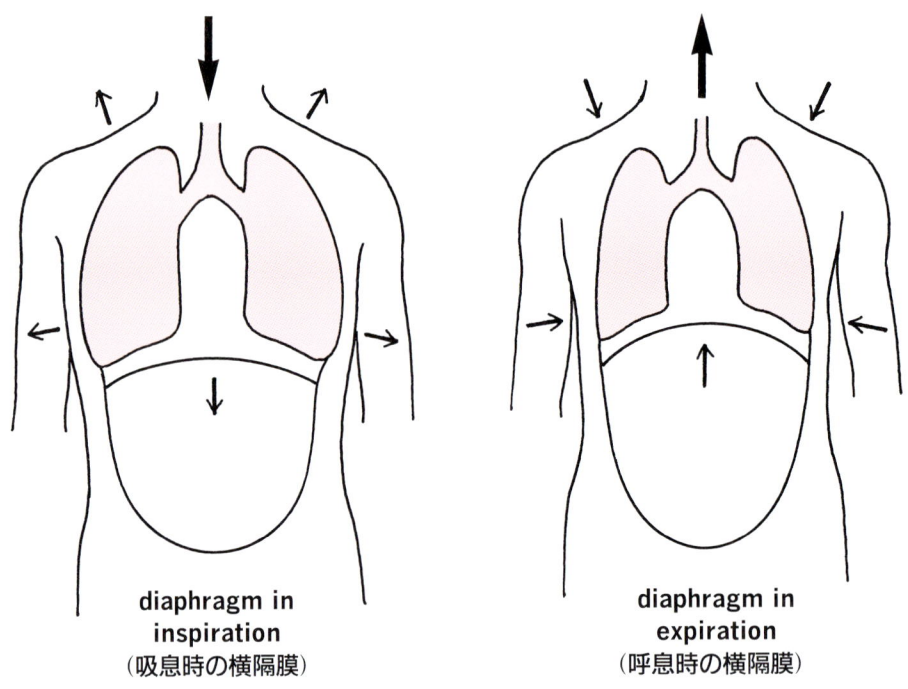

Fig 4-3 Movement of diaphragm

Questions   4(a)

Choose the best word from the list and fill in the blank.

1. The function of the respiratory system is to put _____ into the blood and take out _____.
2. The trachea divides into two big tubes called _____.
3. Each tube goes into the right or left _____ and divides into smaller and smaller tubes called _____.
4. There are very small air sacs called _____ at the end of bronchioles.
5. The _____ is a big muscle under the lungs and above the stomach.

bronchioles	diaphragm	bronchi	alveoli	carbon dioxide
oxygen	lung	trachea		

Chapter 4

Disorders of the Respiratory System
（呼吸器系の疾患）

One of the diseases we often hear about in the respiratory system is called pneumonia. Bacteria go into the different parts of the lungs and make a very bad (acute) infection. Pneumonia is the number one fatal (killing) disease that people get when they stay in the hospital. We breathe in the bad bacteria and they start growing in the bronchioles and then go (spread) to the alveoli and spaces between them. Because of antibiotics like penicillin only about 5% of the people die who get pneumonia. But in America over 2,000,000 people get pneumonia each year. Today, we also have vaccines that help people from getting pneumonia.

Another respiratory disease is called asthma. Some people are very sensitive to things in the air. These things, called irritants, make the muscles of the bronchiole contract and relax quickly. This is called a spasm. The spasm makes the bronchial tubes smaller (narrow) so air cannot go through easily. Therefore, it is difficult to breathe. Instead of making a spasm, the irritant can make the bronchioles get bigger (swell) and make more mucus (a liquid called secretions). This extra mucus blocks the bronchial tubes and it is hard to breathe. Some of the things (irritants) which make (cause) asthma are infections, allergens, cold air, pollution and cigarette smoke.

pneumonia（肺炎）
bacteria（細菌）
acute（急性の）
infection（感染）
fatal（致命的な）
antibiotics（抗生物質）
vaccines（ワクチン）
asthma（喘息）
irritants（刺激物）
contract（収縮する）
relax（弛緩する）
spasm（痙攣）
swell（ふくれる）
mucus（粘液）
secretions（分泌液）
allergens（アレルゲン）
pollution（汚染）

Chapter 4

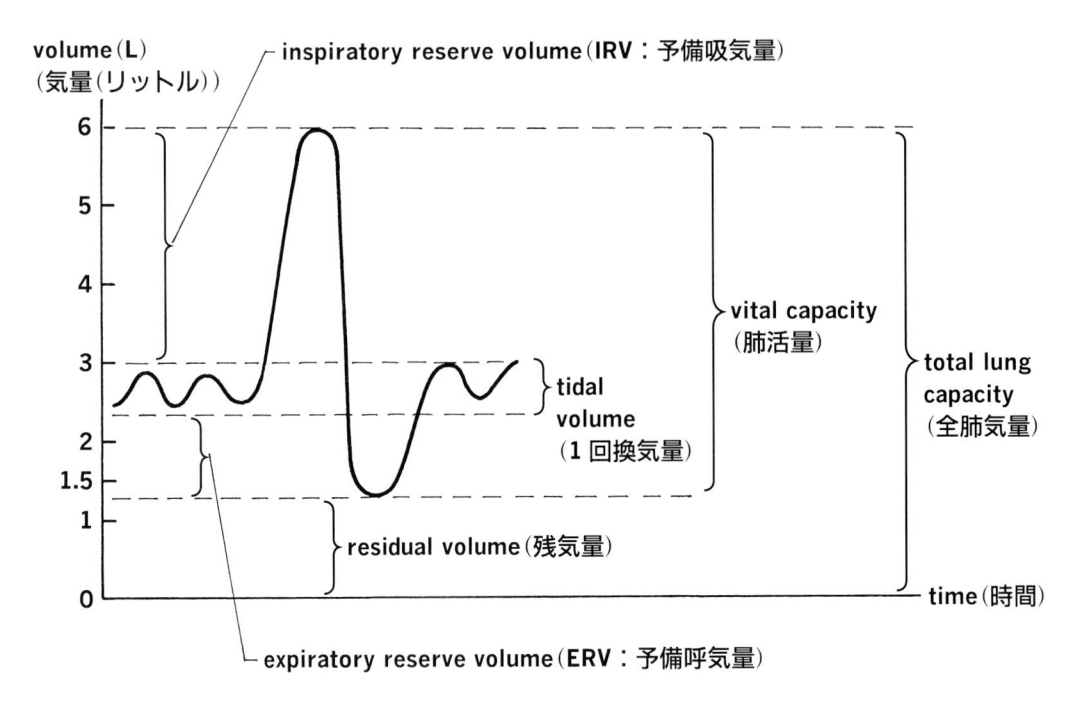

Fig 4-4 Spirogram（スパイログラム）

Questions 4(b)

Choose the best word from the list and fill in the blank.

1. _____ go into the different parts of the lungs and make a very bad (acute) infection.
2. Because of antibiotic medicine like _____ only about 5% of the people die who get pneumonia.
3. Some people are very sensitive to things in the air called _____.
4. The _____ makes the bronchial tubes smaller (narrow) so air can not go through easily.
5. The extra _____ blocks the bronchial tubes and it is hard to breathe.
6. Some of the things which make asthma are infections, _____, cold air, pollution and cigarette smoke.

spasm	bacterium	mucus	penicillin	irritants
allergens	bacteria	pneumonia		

Chapter 4

Vocabulary

rhinitis	鼻炎
pharyngitis	咽頭炎
tonsillitis	扁桃炎
bronchitis	気管支炎
bronchial asthma	気管支喘息
bronchiectasis	気管支拡張症
atelectasis	無気肺
pneumothorax	気胸
pneumonia	肺炎
aspiration pneumonia	誤嚥性肺炎
lobar pneumonia	大葉性肺炎
interstitial pneumonia	間質性肺炎
bacterial pneumonia	細菌性肺炎
fungal pneumonia	真菌性肺炎
pulmonary emphysema	肺気腫
pulmonary tuberculosis	肺結核
pulmonary congestion	肺うっ血
pulmonary edema	肺水腫
pulmonary hemorrhage	肺出血
pulmonary embolism (PE)	肺塞栓
pulmonary infarction	肺梗塞
lung cancer	肺癌
acute lung injury (ALI)	急性肺障害
acute respiratory distress syndrome (ARDS)	急性呼吸窮迫(促迫)症候群
infantile respiratory distress syndrome (IRDS)	新生児呼吸窮迫症候群
chronic obstructive pulmonary disease (COPD)	慢性閉塞性肺疾患
hypoxia	低酸素症
anoxia	酸素欠乏症
hypoxemia	低酸素血症
hypercapnia	高炭酸ガス(症)
asphyxia	窒息

Chapter 4

spirogram	スパイログラム，肺容量曲線
eupnea	正常呼吸
apnea	無呼吸
orthopnea	起座呼吸
dyspnea	呼吸困難
hyperpnea	呼吸亢進，過呼吸
hypopnea	呼吸低下，減呼吸
tachypnea	頻呼吸
bradypnea	徐呼吸
respiratory failure	呼吸不全
Cheyne-Stokes respiration	チェーン・ストークス呼吸

呼吸器系の接頭辞・接尾辞

接頭・接尾	意味	例
a-, an-	無，不，非(not)	anoxia, apnea, atelectasis
brady-	緩徐(slow)	bradypnea
dys-	変質，異常，悪い，困難(bad)	dyspnea
eu-	正常，良好(good)	eupnea
hyper-	過剰，正常範囲を超えている(above, over)	hypercapnia, hyperpnea
hypo-	欠乏，正常以下(under)	hypoxia, hypopnea
ortho-	まっすぐな，直立した	orthopnea
tachy-	急速(quick)	tachypnea
-ectasis	拡張(症)	bronchiectasis, atelectasis
-ia	～症(病気の状態)	hypoxia, anoxia, hypercapnia
-itis	～炎(炎症)	rhinitis, pharyngitis, tonsillitis, bronchitis
-osis	～症(疾病の過程・状況・状態)	tuberculosis
-pnea	呼吸	dyspnea, hyperpnea, hypopnea, tachypnea, bradypnea

Chapter 4

呼吸器系の語根

語根の連結形	意味
rhin/o	鼻(nose)
tonsil/o	扁桃(tonsil)
pharyng/o	咽頭(pharynx, throat)
laryng/o	喉頭(larynx)
trache/o	気管(trachea)
bronch/o	気管支(bronchus)
bronchi/o	気管支(複数形)(bronchi)
pneum/o, pneumon/o, pulm/o, pulmon/o	肺(lung)，気体(gas)，空気(air)
phren/o	横隔膜(diaphragm)
pleur/o	胸膜(pleura)
sin/o, sinus/o	洞，腔(sinus)
spir/o	呼吸(breathing)
steth/o	胸(chest)
thorac/o	胸郭(thorax)
aer/o	空気(air)
pne/o	呼吸(breathing)

練習問題 4

1. **-itis**(〜炎)とつないで次の用語をつくりなさい。

   1 鼻炎 _____ 2 扁桃炎 _____
   3 咽頭炎 _____ 4 喉頭炎 _____
   5 気管炎 _____ 6 気管支炎 _____
   7 横隔膜炎 _____ 8 副鼻腔炎 _____
   9 肺炎 _____ 10 胸膜炎 _____

2. **-pnea**(呼吸)とつないで次の用語をつくりなさい。

   1 無呼吸 _____ 2 呼吸困難 _____
   3 呼吸亢進(過呼吸) _____ 4 呼吸低下(低呼吸) _____
   5 頻呼吸(速呼吸) _____ 6 遅呼吸 _____
   7 起座呼吸 _____ 8 正常呼吸 _____

Chapter 4

3．-stenosis（狭窄）とつないで次の用語をつくりなさい。

1　気管狭窄　＿＿＿＿＿＿＿＿＿　　2　気管支狭窄　＿＿＿＿＿＿＿＿＿

3　胸郭狭窄　＿＿＿＿＿＿＿＿＿　　4　咽頭狭窄　＿＿＿＿＿＿＿＿＿

4．-scope（見るための機器，〜鏡）を含む次の用語の意味をいいなさい。

1　rhinoscope　＿＿＿＿＿＿＿＿＿　　2　pharyngoscope　＿＿＿＿＿＿＿＿＿

3　laryngoscope　＿＿＿＿＿＿＿＿＿　　4　bronchoscope　＿＿＿＿＿＿＿＿＿

5　thoracoscope　＿＿＿＿＿＿＿＿＿　　6　stethoscope　＿＿＿＿＿＿＿＿＿

5．-stomy（開口術）または -tomy（切除，切開術）を含む次の用語の意味をいいなさい。

1　tracheostomy　＿＿＿＿＿＿＿＿＿　　2　tonsillotomy　＿＿＿＿＿＿＿＿＿

3　tracheotomy　＿＿＿＿＿＿＿＿＿　　4　laparotomy　＿＿＿＿＿＿＿＿＿

6．-algia（〜痛）を含む次の用語の意味をいいなさい。

1　rhinalgia　＿＿＿＿＿＿＿＿＿　　2　pharyngalgia　＿＿＿＿＿＿＿＿＿

3　trachealgia　＿＿＿＿＿＿＿＿＿　　4　pleuralgia　＿＿＿＿＿＿＿＿＿

5　thoracalgia　＿＿＿＿＿＿＿＿＿

7．-centesis（穿刺）を含む次の用語の意味をいいなさい。

1　pneumocentesis　＿＿＿＿＿＿＿＿＿　　2　pleurocentesis　＿＿＿＿＿＿＿＿＿

3　thoracocentesis　＿＿＿＿＿＿＿＿＿

8．日本語の意味を調べなさい。

呼吸器系の略語

ALI	acute lung injury	
ARDS	acute respiratory distress syndrome	
ARF	acute respiratory failure	
Bronch	bronchoscopy	
COPD	chronic obstructive pulmonary disease	
CXR	chest X-ray	

DOE	dyspnea on exertion	
ERV	expiratory reserve volume	
IRDS	idiopathic respiratory distress syndrome	
IRDS	infantile respiratory distress syndrome	
IRV	inspiratory reserve volume	
PE	pulmonary embolism	
RV	residual volume	
SARS	severe acute respiratory syndrome	
SOB	shortness of breath	
SOBE	shortness of breath on exertion	
TB	tuberculosis	
TLC	total lung capacity	
TV	tidal volume	
URI	upper respiratory infection	
URTI	upper respiratory tract infection	
VC	vital capacity	

Chapter 5

Digestive System
（消化器系）

Overview

The digestive tract is like a long tube that begins at the mouth and ends at the anus. Food moves from the mouth through the esophagus to the stomach and then into the small intestine and then into the large intestine and finally into the rectum and out through the anus. Digestion means to break up the food into small pieces, called nutrients, so they can pass into the blood and go to all the parts of the body. The digestive tract has muscles that move food like a wave. We call this action peristalsis.

The organs of the digestive system like the mouth, stomach, pancreas and liver make special substances which break up the food into nutrients. These special substances are called enzymes. The gallbladder is an organ attached to the liver and it stores a special fluid called bile. This helps to digest the fatty parts of food.

The inside wall of the digestive tract has a special covering called the lining. The lining is where the nutrients actually pass from the tract into the blood. The blood from the intestines flows to the liver, carrying nutrients, vitamins, minerals and other products from digestion.

- digestive tract（消化管）
- anus（肛門）
- stomach（胃）
- intestine（腸）
- rectum（直腸）
- digestion（消化）
- nutrients（栄養物）
- peristalsis（蠕動運動）
- pancreas（膵臓）
- liver（肝臓）
- substances（物質）
- enzyme（酵素）
- gallbladder（胆嚢）
- fluid（液体）
- bile（胆汁）
- fatty（脂肪の）
- lining（内張）

Chapter 5

The liver, which is the biggest organ of the body, does more than 200 jobs. It stores some nutrients, changes them from one form to another, and releases them into the blood according to the activities and needs of the body. Finally, anything that was not digested in the small intestine such as spare water and body minerals, is absorbed through the walls of the large intestine, and goes back into the blood. The parts of the food which we never need, or things that the body used up, become feces. The feces are stored in the rectum and are finally squeezed through a ring of muscle called the anus, and out of the body.

release（放出する）

mineral（無機物）

absorb（吸収する）

feces（糞便）

squeeze（絞り出す）

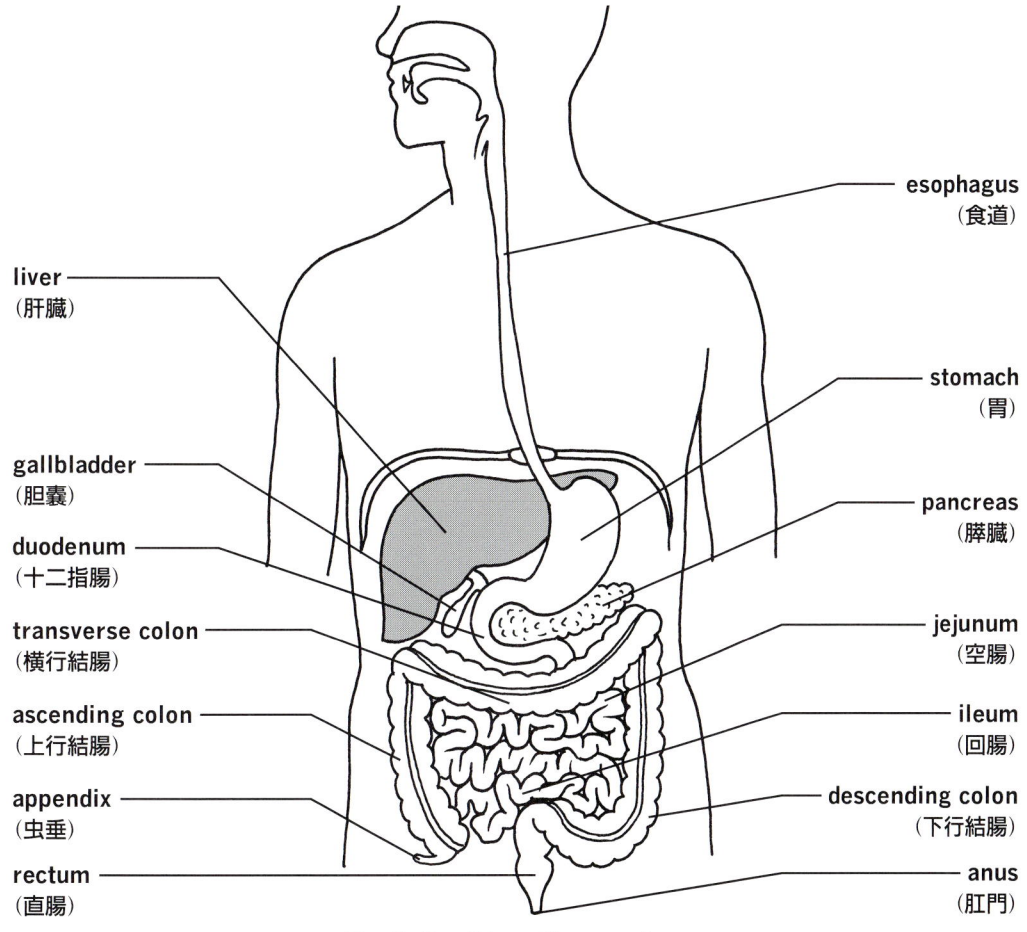

Fig 5-1 Digestive system

- liver（肝臓）
- gallbladder（胆嚢）
- duodenum（十二指腸）
- transverse colon（横行結腸）
- ascending colon（上行結腸）
- appendix（虫垂）
- rectum（直腸）
- esophagus（食道）
- stomach（胃）
- pancreas（膵臓）
- jejunum（空腸）
- ileum（回腸）
- descending colon（下行結腸）
- anus（肛門）

Chapter 5

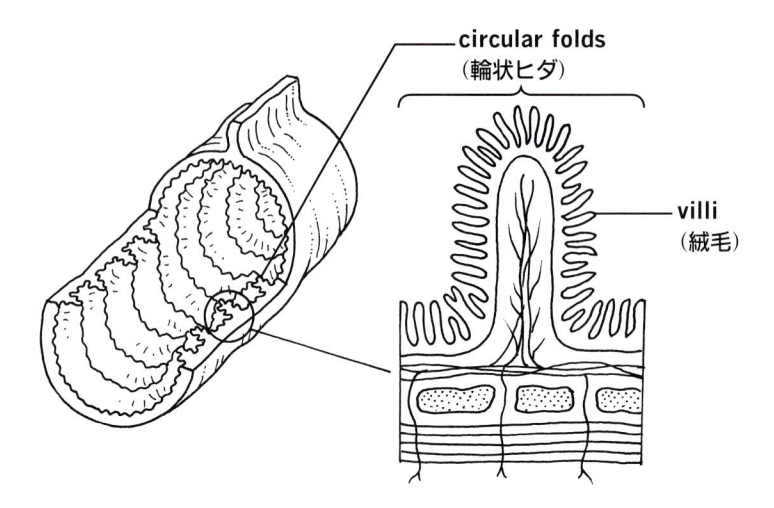

Fig 5-2 Internal structure of small intestine

Questions 5(a)

Choose the best word from the list and fill in the blank.

1. The digestive tract begins at the _____ and ends at the _____.
2. Food moves from the mouth through the _____ to the stomach.
3. The digestive tract move food like a wave. We call this _____.
4. Some digestive organs make special substances called _____.
5. The _____ stores a special chemical called bile.
6. The bile helps to digest _____ parts of food.
7. The inside of the walls of the digestive tract is called the _____.
8. The _____ is the biggest organ of the body and does more than 200 jobs.

| anus | gallbladder | mouth | pancreas | liver | esophagus |
| nutrient | enzymes | fatty | peristalsis | lining | |

Chapter 5

Disorders of the Digestive System
(消化器系の疾患)

The word *peptic* means digestive so we are talking about peptic ulcers. A peptic ulcer is a sore on the lining of the stomach or duodenum. One cause of peptic ulcer is bacterial infection but some ulcers are caused by long-term use of nonsteroidal anti-inflammatory agents (NSAIDs), like aspirin and ibuprofen. Ulcers are not caused by spicy food or stress, but they may make them worse.

Doctors believe that the bacterium *Helicobacter pylori* (*H. pylori*) is responsible for most peptic ulcers. In Japan about fifty percent, in other Asian countries about eighty percent and in the U.S. about 25 percent of people are infected with *H. pylori*. However, most infected people do not get ulcers. It is not certain how people get *H. pylori*, but it may be through food or water.

Nowadays, *H. pylori* peptic ulcers are effectively treated with a combination of drugs. Antibiotics kill the bacteria and other drugs reduce the gastric acid and protect the lining of stomach.

Viral hepatitis is a common disease. That makes the liver become inflamed. There are more than six different viruses

---

peptic（消化性の）

ulcer（潰瘍）

sore（びらん）

lining（内張り）

duodenum（十二指腸）

non-steroidal anti-inflammatory agents（非ステロイド性抗炎症剤）

aspirin（アスピリン）

ibuprofen（イブプロフェン）

Helicobacter pylori, H. pylori（ヘリコバクター・ピロリ，ピロリ菌）

effectively（有効に）

antibiotics（抗生物質）

gastric acid（胃酸）

viral hepatitis（ウイルス性肝炎）
inflamed（炎症をおこした）

Chapter 5

which cause hepatitis. Three of them, hepatitis A virus (HAV), hepatitis B virus (HBV) and hepatitis C virus (HCV) have been studied well. Hepatitis A which is caused by HAV comes from infected foods and causes fever and jaundice. Hepatitis B which is caused by HBV is a severe form and is transmitted by infected blood. It causes fever, debility and jaundice. Hepatitis C which is caused by HCV is also transmitted by infected blood. Hepatitis B and C sometimes develop chronic hepatitis, then cirrhosis, and finally cancer. We can protect against Hepatitis B by vaccine but there is no vaccine for Hepatitis C.

fever（発熱）
jaundice（黄疸）
transmit（伝染させる）
infect（感染する）
debility（衰弱）
chronic（慢性の）
cirrhosis（肝硬変）
cancer（癌）
vaccine（ワクチン）

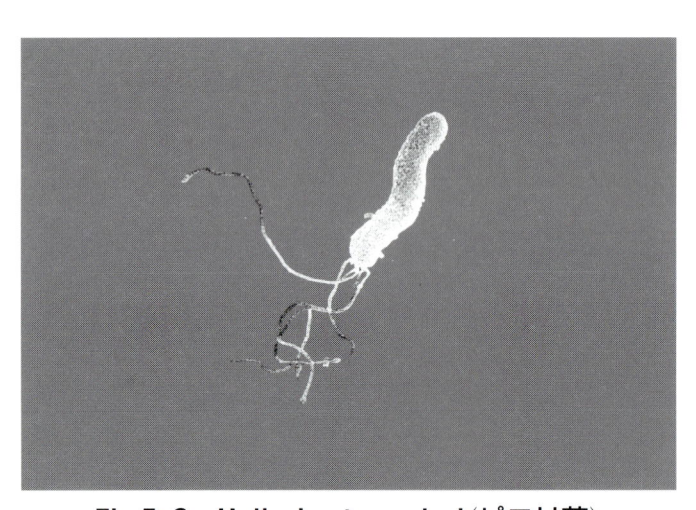

Fig 5-3　Helicobacter pylori（ピロリ菌）
（井上泰：学生のための疾病論，医学書院，2001，p.89 掲載の新
　潟大学細菌学教室　山本達男教授提供の写真より）

Chapter 5

Questions 5(b)

Choose the best word from the list and fill in the blank.

1. Some peptic ulcers are caused by drugs like _____.
2. The _____ called *H. pylori* is responsible for most peptic ulcers.
3. Hepatitis A comes from _____ infected with HAV.
4. HBV and HCV are transmitted by tainted _____.
5. We can protect against Hepatitis B by _____.
6. Hepatitis C can develop chronic hepatitis, then _____ and finally _____.

| vaccine | bacterium | blood | aspirin | food | antibiotics |
| cancer | jaundice | cirrhosis | | | |

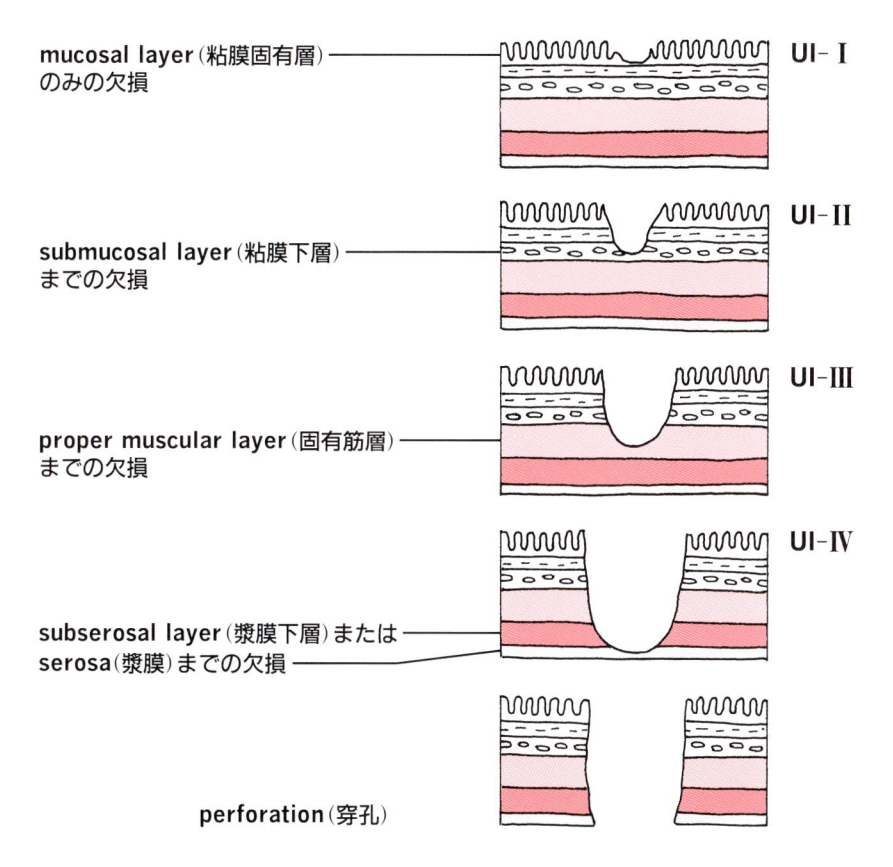

---

mucosal layer(粘膜固有層)のみの欠損 — UI-I

submucosal layer(粘膜下層)までの欠損 — UI-II

proper muscular layer(固有筋層)までの欠損 — UI-III

subserosal layer(漿膜下層)または serosa(漿膜)までの欠損 — UI-IV

perforation(穿孔)

Fig 5-4　Classification of gastric ulcers(胃潰瘍の深さによる分類)

Chapter 5

Vocabulary

oral cancer	口腔癌
achalasia	アカラジア(特発性食道拡張症)
esophageal varix	食道静脈瘤
gastritis	胃炎
gastric ulcer (GU)	胃潰瘍
peptic ulcer (PU)	消化性潰瘍
gastric polyp	胃ポリープ
gastric carcinoma	胃癌
hypertrophic pyloric stenosis	肥厚性幽門狭窄(症)
duodenal ulcer (DU)	十二指腸潰瘍
Crohn's disease (CD)	クローン病
ulcerative colitis (UC)	潰瘍性大腸炎
bacillary dysentery	細菌性赤痢
appendicitis	虫垂炎
ileus	腸閉塞(イレウス)
hernia	ヘルニア
tumor of colon	大腸腫瘍
carcinoma of colon	大腸癌
colorectal cancer	結腸・直腸がん
peritonitis	腹膜炎
jaundice	黄疸
viral hepatitis	ウイルス性肝炎
fatty liver	脂肪肝
liver cirrhosis	肝硬変
hepatic encephalopathy	肝性脳症
liver carcinoma (hepatoma)	肝臓癌
gallstone	胆石
cholelithiasis (cholecystolithiasis)	胆石症
pancreatitis	膵炎
pancreatic carcinoma	膵癌
dysphagia (dysphagy)	嚥下困難(障害)
maldigestion (dyspepsia)	消化不良

malabsorption		吸収不良
constipation		便秘(症)
diarrhea		下痢

接頭辞・接尾辞

接頭・接尾	意味	例
dys-	変質，異常，悪い，困難(eu- の対語)	dyspepsia, dysphagia
mal-	悪い，不良(eu- の対語)	maldigestion, malabsorption
-itis	～炎(炎症)	appendicitis, colitis, gastritis, hepatitis, pancreatitis, peritonitis
-ia	～症(病気の状態)	dyspepsia, dysphagia, hernia
-iasis	～症(不健康な状態)	cholelithiasis, cholecystolithiasis
-oma	腫瘍，新生物	hepatoma
-osis	～症(疾病の過程・状況・状態)	cirrhosis
-phage, -phagia, -phagy	食べる	dysphagia, dysphagy

消化器系の語根

語根の連結形	意味
or/o, stomat/o	口(mouth)
dent/i, odont/o	歯(teeth)
pharyng/o	咽頭(pharynx)
esophag/o	食道(esophagus)
gastr/o	胃(stomach)
duoden/o	十二指腸(duodenum)
enter/o	小腸(small intestine)
pylor/o	幽門(pylorus, pl. pylori)
jejun/o	空腸(jejunum)
ile/o	回腸(ileum)

Chapter 5

語根の連結形	意味
cec/o	盲腸 (cecum)
col/o, colon/o	大腸 (colon, large intestine)
sigmoid/o	S 字状結腸 (sigmoid colon)
rect/o	直腸 (rectum)
an/o, proct/o	肛門 (anus)
hepat/o	肝臓 (liver)
pancreat/o	膵臓 (pancreas)
cholecyst/o	胆嚢 (gallbladder)
chol/o	胆汁 (bile)
lith/o	石 (stone)
peritone/o	腹膜 (peritoneum)

練習問題 5

1. -itis（～炎）とつないで次の用語をつくりなさい。
   1. 口内炎　＿＿＿＿＿＿＿　　2. 食道炎　＿＿＿＿＿＿＿
   3. 胃炎　＿＿＿＿＿＿＿　　4. 膵炎　＿＿＿＿＿＿＿
   5. 胃腸炎　＿＿＿＿＿＿＿　　6. 小腸炎　＿＿＿＿＿＿＿
   7. 大腸炎（結腸炎）＿＿＿＿＿＿＿　　8. 虫垂炎　＿＿＿＿＿＿＿
   9. 腹膜炎　＿＿＿＿＿＿＿　　10. 肛門周囲炎　＿＿＿＿＿＿＿

2. -algia（～痛）とつないで次の用語をつくりなさい。
   1. 歯痛　＿＿＿＿＿＿＿　　2. 胃痛　＿＿＿＿＿＿＿
   3. 咽頭痛　＿＿＿＿＿＿＿　　4. 肛門痛　＿＿＿＿＿＿＿

3. hepat-（肝臓）を含む次の用語の意味をいいなさい。
   1. hepatitis　＿＿＿＿＿＿＿　　2. hepatomegaly　＿＿＿＿＿＿＿
   3. hepatoma　＿＿＿＿＿＿＿　　4. hepatatrophy　＿＿＿＿＿＿＿
   5. hepatectomy　＿＿＿＿＿＿＿　　6. hepatic　＿＿＿＿＿＿＿

Chapter 5

4．次の用語の意味をいいなさい。
　　1　acute gastritis _____　　2　chronic gastritis _____
　　3　early gastric carcinoma _____
　　4　advanced gastric carcinoma _____

5．jejuno-(空腸)を含む次の用語の意味をいいなさい。
　　1　jejunostomy _____
　　2　jejunojejunostomy _____
　　3　jejunotomy _____　　4　jejunectomy _____

6．colo-(大腸)を含む次の用語の意味をいいなさい。
　　1　colostomy _____　　2　colotomy _____
　　3　coloproctostomy _____　　4　colectomy _____

7．次の用語の意味をいいなさい。
　　1　cholecystectomy _____　　2　laparoscopy _____
　　3　laparoscopic cholecystectomy(LC) _____
　　4　polypectomy _____
　　5　colonoscopic polypectomy _____
　　6　peritoneocentesis _____

8．日本語の意味を調べなさい。

消化器系の略語

Abdo	abdomen	
CD	Crohn's disease	
DU	duodenal ulcer	
EMR	endoscopic mucosal resection	
ERCP	endoscopic retrograde cholangiopancreatography	
GB	gallbladder	
GI	gastrointestinal	

Chapter 5

G-I series	gastro-intestinal series	
GU	gastric ulcer	
HA	hepatitis A	
HAV	hepatitis A virus	
HB	hepatitis B	
HCC	hepatocellular carcinoma	
HCV	hepatitis C virus	
IBS	irritable bowel syndrome	
IUC	idiopathic ulcerative colitis	
pr, PR	per rectum	
PU	peptic ulcer	
RE	rectal examination	
UC	ulcerative colitis	
UGI	upper gastrointestinal series	
VF	videofluorography	

病院の診療科と診察医

診療科名および診察医に関する次の表を完成しなさい。

Department of medicine	診療科名	Doctors
internal medicine	内科	internist
cardiology		
pulmonary medicine		
gastroenterology		
endocrinology		
psychosomatic medicine		
surgery		
orthopedics		
neurosurgery		
plastic surgery		
obstetrics		
gynecology		
pediatrics		
psychiatry		
neurology		
urology		
dermatology		
ophthalmology		
otorhinolaryngology ENT(Ear, Nose, Throat)		
dentistry		
radiology		
anesthesiology		

Chapter 6

Urinary System
（泌尿器系）

Overview

The urinary system includes two kidneys, two ureters, the bladder, two sphincter muscles, and the urethra. The function (job) of the urinary system is to remove liquid wastes (bad things) from the blood. The lungs, skin and intestines also excrete wastes from the body. All these systems keep the chemicals and water in your body balanced.

The main part of the urinary system is the kidney. We have two kidneys. They are bean-shaped organs about the size of your fists. They are near the middle of the back, just below the rib cage. Each kidney has many very small filters called nephrons. A nephron is like a ball made of small blood capillaries. This ball part is called a *glomerulus*. The other part of the nephron is a small tube called a renal tubule.

Urea, together with water and other waste substances, forms the urine. This passes through the nephrons and down the renal tubules of the kidney.

Each kidney has a tube called a ureter that carries urine to a storage bag called a bladder. When the bladder is filled up,

---

kidney（腎臓）
ureter（尿管）
bladder（膀胱）
sphincter muscle（括約筋）
urethra（尿道）
waste（老廃物）
excrete（排泄する）
chemical（化学物質）
bean-shaped（そら豆の形をした）
fist（握りこぶし）
rib（肋骨）
filter（濾過器）
nephron（ネフロン）
glomerulus（糸球体）
renal tubule（尿細管）
urea（尿素）
substance（物質）
urine（尿）

Chapter 6

special muscles in the bladder contract (squeeze). This pushes the urine out of our body through a tube called a urethra. When the urine comes out of our body we call it urination. Each day our kidneys make about 1.5 liters of urine.

Healthy kidneys also control blood pressure, keep bones strong and tell your body to make red blood cells.

contract（収縮する）

urination（排尿）

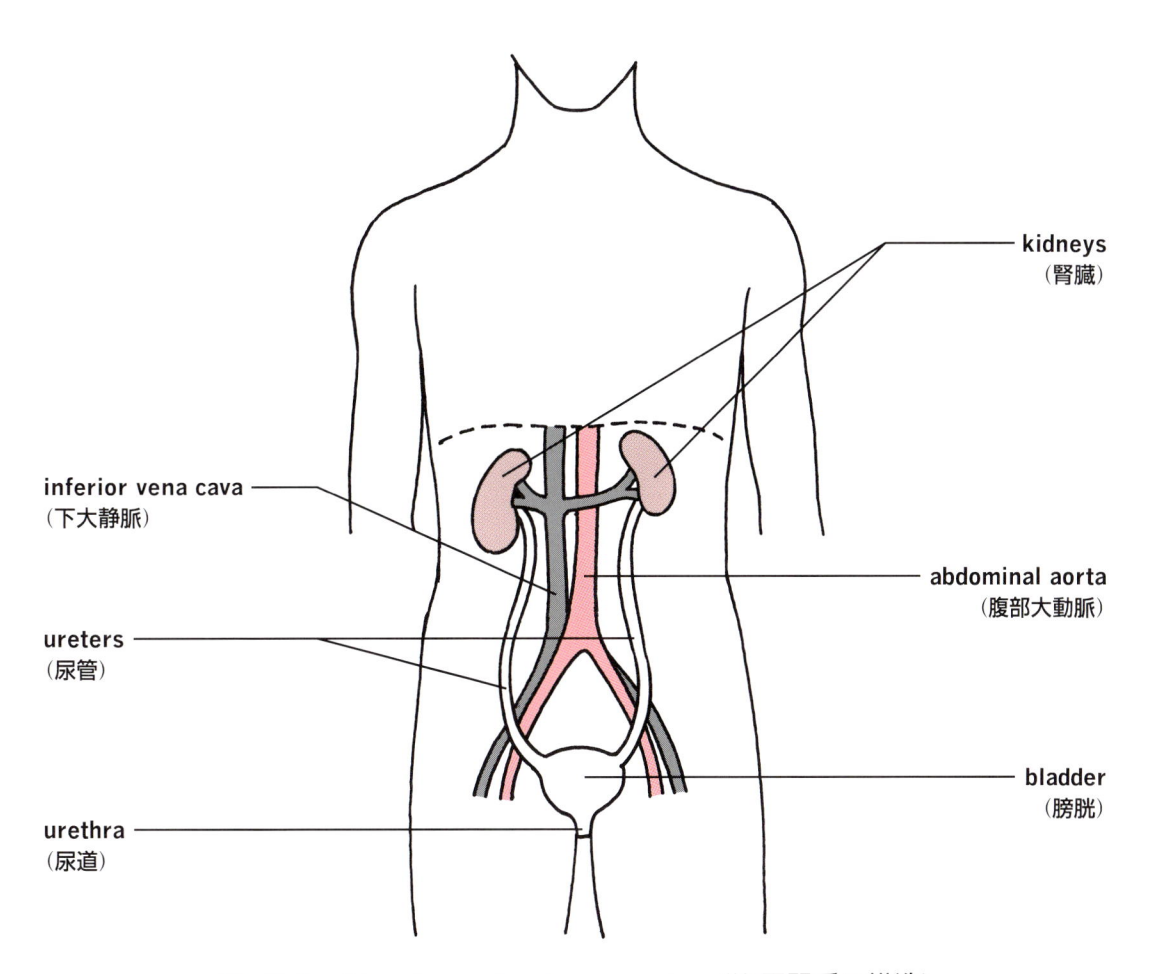

Fig 6-1　Structure of urinary system（泌尿器系の構造）

- kidneys（腎臓）
- inferior vena cava（下大静脈）
- abdominal aorta（腹部大動脈）
- ureters（尿管）
- bladder（膀胱）
- urethra（尿道）

Chapter 6

Questions 6(a)

Choose the best word from the list and fill in the blank.

1. The function of the urinary system is to remove liquid _____ from the blood.
2. The main part of the urinary system is the _____.
3. Kidneys are bean-shaped organs about the size of your _____.
4. Each kidney has many very small filters called _____.
5. The kidneys make a liquid called _____.
6. There is a tube going out of each kidney called a _____.
7. Urine comes out of our body through a tube called a _____.

urine	urethra	nephrons	glomerulus	kidney	fists
ureter	wastes	urea			

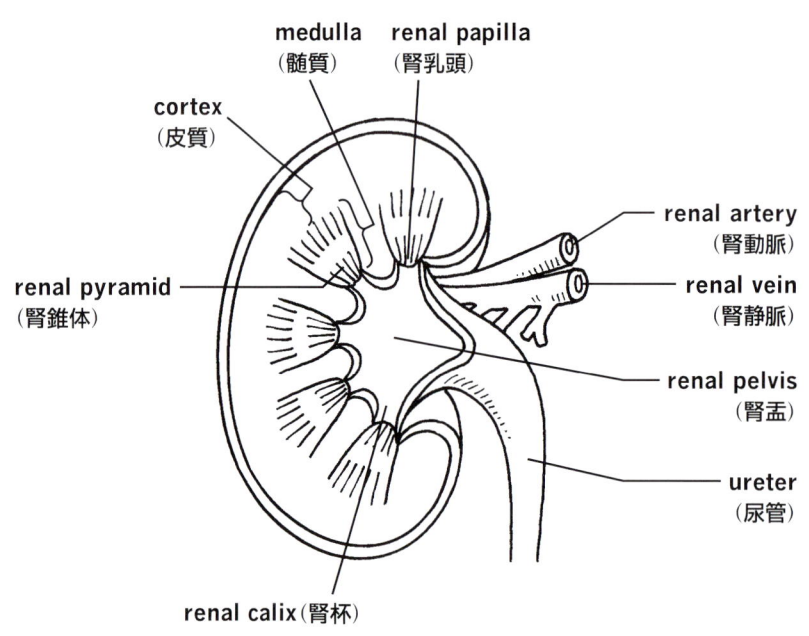

Fig 6-2 Sectional figure of kidney (腎臓の断面図)

Chapter 6

Disorders of the Urinary System
（泌尿器系の疾患）

Remember that the kidneys are the most important part of the urinary system. The word *renes* means kidney and the adjective form of the word is renal.

renal（腎臓の）

One of the most serious disorders of the urinary system is renal failure (kidneys stop working). Healthy kidneys remove extra water and wastes, help control blood pressure, keep body chemicals in balance, keep bones strong and tell your body to make red blood cells.

renal failure（腎不全）
extra（余剰の）
wastes（老廃物）

There are two types of renal failure: acute and chronic. Acute renal failure (ARF) means it occurs suddenly and is very bad.

acute（急性の）
chronic（慢性の）

People can get acute renal failure from a toxin (a drug allergy) or much bleeding after surgery. Dialysis is used to clean the blood and give the kidneys a rest. If the cause is treated, the kidneys may be able to recover some or all of their functions.

bleeding（出血）
dialysis（血液透析）
treat（治療する）

The other kind of renal failure is called chronic renal failure (CRF). The kidneys become weaker and stop doing their work slowly over a long period of time. This type of problem can be caused by chronic glomerulonephritis, diabetic nephro-

glomerulonephritis
（糸球体腎炎）
diabetic nephropathy
（糖尿病性腎症）
nephrosclerosis
（腎硬化症）

Chapter 6

pathy, nephrosclerosis, and polycystic kidney. Most people with chronic renal failure develop a condition called end-stage renal failure (ESRF). This can be treated by dialysis or by a kidney transplant. Dialysis is effective, but it is not a 'cure' and may not get rid of all the symptoms. A successful kidney transplant is a more effective treatment than dialysis. However, it is not easy to find a compatible donor kidney.

| polycystic kidney（多発性嚢胞腎） |
| end-stage（終末期） |
| transplant（移植） |
| cure（治療） |
| symptoms（症状） |
| compatible（適合性のある） |
| donor（提供者） |

chronic renal failure
（慢性腎不全）
表面凹凸
萎縮

normal kidney
（正常腎）
表面平滑

acute renal failure
（急性腎不全）
表面平滑緊満
腫大

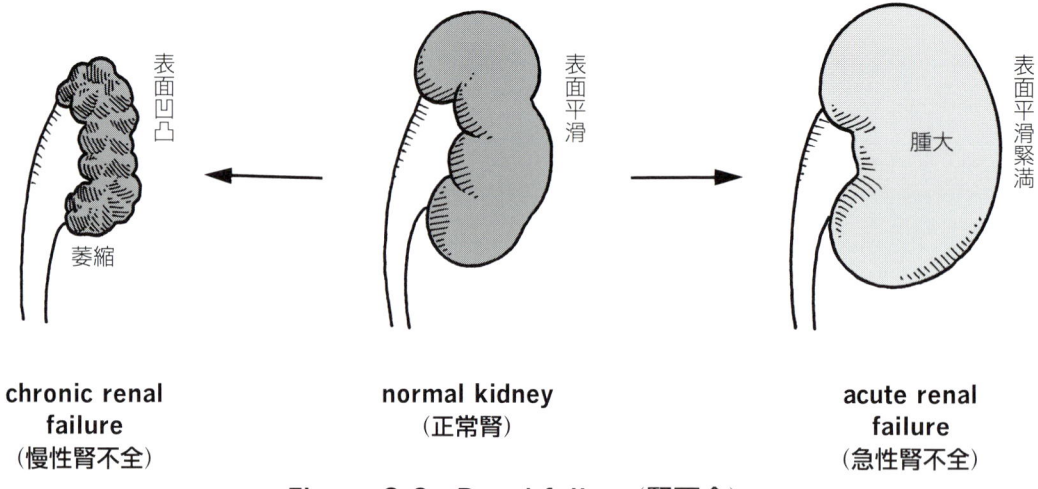

Figure 6-3　Renal failure（腎不全）

Questions 6(b)

Choose the best word from the list and fill in the blank.

1. The doctors who take care of the urinary system are called ＿＿＿＿.
2. One of the most serious disorders of the urinary system is ＿＿＿＿.
3. Kidneys will keep the right water ＿＿＿＿ in the tissues.
4. There are two types of renal failure, ＿＿＿＿ and chronic.
5. Chronic renal failure can be caused by ＿＿＿＿.
6. The treatment of end-stage renal failure is either ＿＿＿＿ or kidney transplant.

```
acute      dialysis      urologists      balance      renal failure
chronic  glomerulonephritis
```

52

Chapter 6

Vocabulary

renal failure	腎不全
acute renal failure (ARF)	急性腎不全
chronic renal failure (CRF)	慢性腎不全
tubular necrosis	尿細管壊死
glomerulonephritis	糸球体腎炎
pyelonephritis	腎盂腎炎
nephroblastoma	腎芽細胞腫
nephrosclerosis	腎硬化症
nephrotic syndrome	ネフローゼ症候群
diabetic nephropathy	糖尿病性腎症
radiocontrast nepropathy	造影剤腎症
IgA nephropathy	IgA 腎症
hydronephrosis	水腎症
lupus nephritis	ループス腎炎
amyloidosis	アミロイドーシス
hemolytic uremic syndrome(HUS)	溶血性尿毒症症候群
cystitis	膀胱炎
polycystic kidney	多発性嚢胞腎
renal infarction	腎梗塞
renal vein thrombosis	腎静脈血栓症
renal hypertension	腎性高血圧
renal calculus (calculi)	腎結石
urinary calculus (calculi)	尿路結石
urinary tract infection (UTI)	尿路感染症
uremia	尿毒症
ureteritis	尿管炎
urethritis	尿道炎
polyuria	多尿(症)
oliguria	乏尿(症)
dysuria	排尿困難

Chapter 6

isch**uria**		尿閉
incontinence of urine		尿失禁

接頭辞・接尾辞

接頭・接尾	意味	例
dys-	困難，不良，悪い，異常	dysuria
-emia	〜血症(血液中に〜の存在する状態)	uremia
-iasis	〜症(不健康な状態)	urolithiasis
-itis	〜炎(炎症)	nephritis, ureteritis, cystitis
-oma	腫瘍，新生物	nephroblastoma
-osis	〜症(疾病の過程，状況，状態)	hydronephrosis, necrosis nephrosclerosis
-pathy	〜症，〜療法	nephropathy
-uria	〜尿症(尿中に〜の存在する状態)	dysuria, ischuria, oliguria, polyuria

泌尿器系の語根

語根の連結形	意味
ren/o, nephr/o	腎臓(kidney)
pyel/o	腎盂(pelvis)
ureter/o	尿管(ureter)
cyst/o	膀胱(bladder)
urethr/o	尿道(urethra)
uri/a, urin/o, urin/i	尿(urine)
ur/o	尿，排尿(urine, micturition)
lith/o	石(stone)
glomerul/o	糸球体(glomerulus)

Chapter 6

練習問題 6

1. -itis（～炎）とつないで次の用語をつくりなさい。
   1　腎炎　_____　　2　糸球体腎炎　_____
   3　腎盂炎　_____　　4　尿管炎　_____
   5　膀胱炎　_____　　6　尿道炎　_____

2. -uria（～尿症）とつないで次の用語をつくりなさい。
   1　蛋白尿症　_____　　2　排尿困難　_____
   3　多尿症　_____　　4　乏尿症　_____

3. -lith（～結石）とつないで次の用語をつくりなさい。
   1　腎結石　_____　　2　腎盂結石　_____
   3　尿管結石　_____　　4　膀胱結石　_____

4. -uria（～尿症）を含む次の用語の意味をいいなさい。
   1　glycosuria（glucosuria）_____
   2　albuminuria　_____　　3　azoturia　_____
   4　hematuria　_____

5. -ostomy（造ろう術，吻合術）を含む次の用語の意味をいいなさい。
   1　pyelostomy　_____　　2　ureterostomy　_____
   3　urethrostomy　_____　　4　urethrocystostomy　_____

6. 日本語の意味を調べなさい。

泌尿器系の略語

ADH	antidiuretic hormone	
AGN	acute glomerulonephritis	
ARF	acute renal failure	
BUN	blood urea nitrogen	
CGN	chronic glomerulonephritis	

Chapter 6

Ccr	creatinine clearance	
CRF	chronic renal failure	
CYS	cystoscopy	
ESRF	end-stage renal failure	
GFR	glomerular filtration rate	
HD	hemodialysis	
HUS	hemolytic uremic syndrome	
IVP	intravenous pyelogram	
IVU	intravenous urogram	
KUB	kidney, ureter and bladder	
UA	urine analysis	
U&E	urea and electrolytes	
UAE	urine albumin excretion	
UG	urogenital	
ur	urine	
UTI	urinary tract infection	

痛みの表現

a _____ pain

種類	slow dull	シクシクする
	prickling	チクチクする
	tingling	ヒリヒリする
	stinging	ズキズキ刺すような
	throbbing	ずきんずきんという
	stabbing	グサリと刺すような
	racking	(拷問にかけられるような)ひどい
程度	slight	軽い
	moderate	中くらいの
	unbearable (untolerable)	我慢できない
	severe	激しい
	dull	鈍い
	sharp	鋭い
持続期間	sudden	突然の
	gradual	徐々にでてくる
	occasional	時折の
	intermittent	間欠的な
	constant	持続的な
	persistent	持続的な
	chronic	慢性の

Chapter 7

Nervous System
（神経系）

Overview

The nervous system is the most important of the body's systems. It lets us move and feel things. The brain is the biggest and main part of the nervous system (NS). The smallest part of the NS is a cell, called a neuron. The brain has about 100 billion neurons. A nerve is a collection (group) of neurons that communicate with each other by chemicals, called neurotransmitters. Many nerves leave the brain and go down the middle of the back (spine). This is like the trunk of a tree. The nerves in the brain and spinal cord are called the central nervous system (CNS).

From the brain and spinal cord other nerves go out like branches. These branches keep dividing and get smaller until they reach every part of our body. All the nerves after the brain and spinal cord are called the peripheral nervous system (PNS). Peripheral means on the outside, not in the center. All nerves work in pairs. One part carries information from the brain and lets us move muscles to control our body movements. These are called motor nerves. The other nerves sends messages to the brain and lets us feel things (see, hear, smell, taste, and touch). These are sensory

---

brain（脳）

billion（10億）
neuron（ニューロン）
nerve（神経）
communicate（連絡する）
chemicals（化学物質）
neurotransmitters
（神経伝達物質）
spine（脊椎）
spinal cord（脊髄）
central nervous system
（中枢神経系）
branches（枝）
peripheral nervous system
（末梢神経系）

information（情報）
control（支配する）
movements（動き）
motor nerves（運動神経）

Chapter 7

nerves.

Voluntary nerves are the motor nerves we can control by thinking. But some nerves work without our thinking. We don't think of breathing or peristaltic movement of stomach and intestine. These nerves are called involuntary nerves.

sensory nerves(感覚神経)

voluntary nerves(随意神経)

peristaltic(ぜん動の)

involuntary nerves(不随意神経)

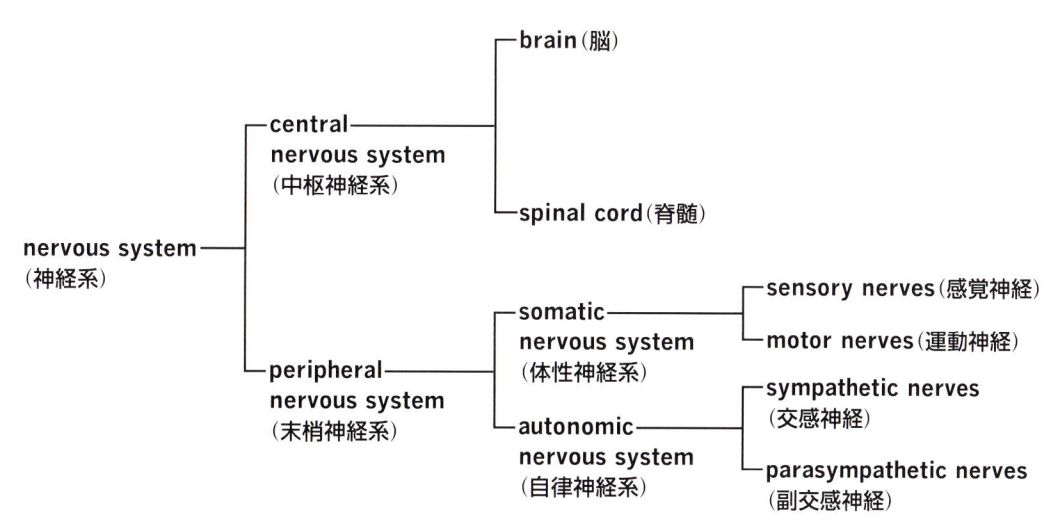

Fig 7-1　神経系の構成（Nervous system）

- nervous system（神経系）
  - central nervous system（中枢神経系）
    - brain（脳）
    - spinal cord（脊髄）
  - peripheral nervous system（末梢神経系）
    - somatic nervous system（体性神経系）
      - sensory nerves（感覚神経）
      - motor nerves（運動神経）
    - autonomic nervous system（自律神経系）
      - sympathetic nerves（交感神経）
      - parasympathetic nerves（副交感神経）

Chapter 7

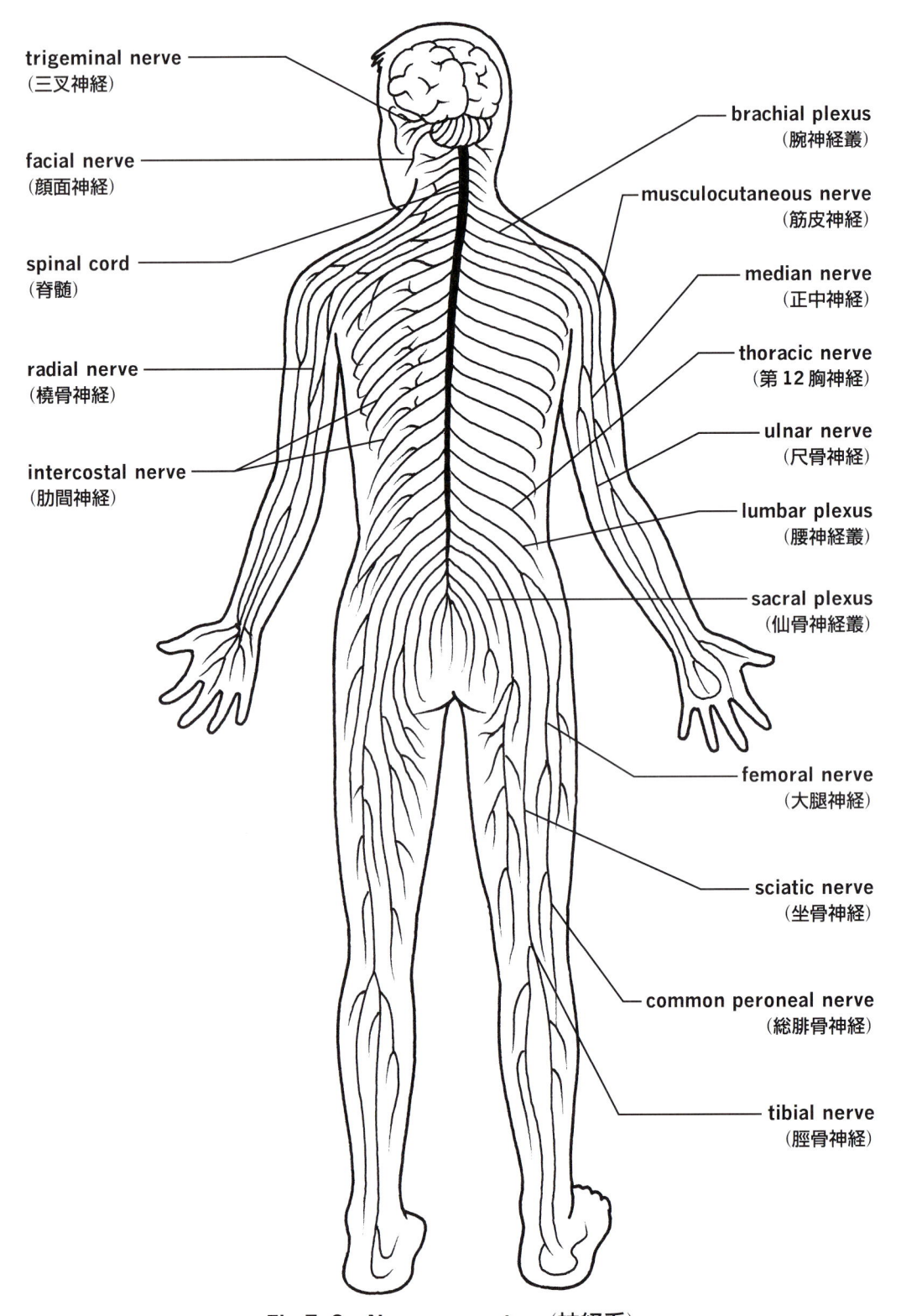

Fig 7-2 Nervous system（神経系）

Chapter 7

Questions 7(a)

Choose the best word from the list and fill in the blank.

1. The brain is the biggest and main part of the _____ system.
2. The brain has over 100 billion _____.
3. The nerves in the brain and _____ cord are called the central nervous system (CNS).
4. Peripheral means on the _____, not in the center.
5. One part of a nerve carries information from the brain and lets us move muscles to control our body movements. These are called _____ nerves.
6. The nerves we can control by thinking are called _____ nerves.

outside	inside	motor	voluntary	involuntary
nervous	neurons	spinal		

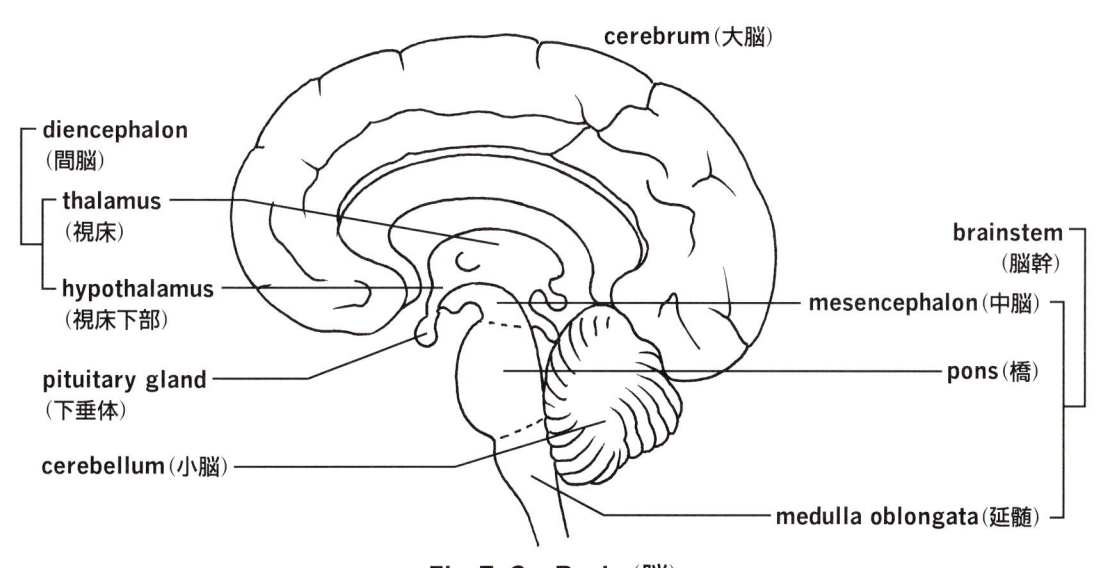

Fig 7-3 Brain(脳)

Chapter 7

Disorders of the Nervous System
（神経系の疾患）

When there is not enough blood going to parts of the brain we get a stroke. Brain cells are very sensitive and if they don't get enough food and oxygen for a few minutes they will die.

Different parts of the brain take care of different things that we do. The back part of the brain (occipital lobe) takes care of seeing. The left side is for language and the front part is for thinking. Sometimes only small blood vessels (tubes) are blocked and the part of the brain that they go to will have only a small effect. Maybe the fingers of one hand will not work (paralysis). But sometimes a big blood vessel is blocked and many brain cells (neurons) die. Then the patient may develop paralysis on one or both sides of the body; have difficulty in walking, eating, or other daily activities. Maybe they will not be able to speak nor understand speech.

Parkinson's disease is a progressive neurological disorder. The disease results from degeneration of neurons in a region of the brain that controls movement. This degeneration causes a shortage of the neurotransmitter called dopamine. This lack of dopamine causes the movement problems that we see in Parkinson's patients.

---

stroke（脳卒中）

occipital lobe（後頭葉）

paralysis（麻痺）

progressive（進行性の）
neurological disorder（神経疾患）
degeneration（変性）
movement（運動）
causes（引き起こす）
shortage（不足）

Chapter 7

The first sign of Parkinson's disease is tremor (trembling or shaking) of a limb, especially when the body is at rest. Other common signs include slow movement (bradykinesia), an inability to move (akinesia), rigid limbs, a shuffling gait, and a stooped posture. L-Dopa is one medicine that can help some people with Parkinson's disease.

sign（徴候）
tremor（振戦）
limb（手足）
bradykinesia（動作緩慢）
inability（不能）
akinesia（無運動）
rigid（硬直した）
shuffling（足をひきずる）
gait（歩行）
stooped（前かがみになった）
posture（姿勢）

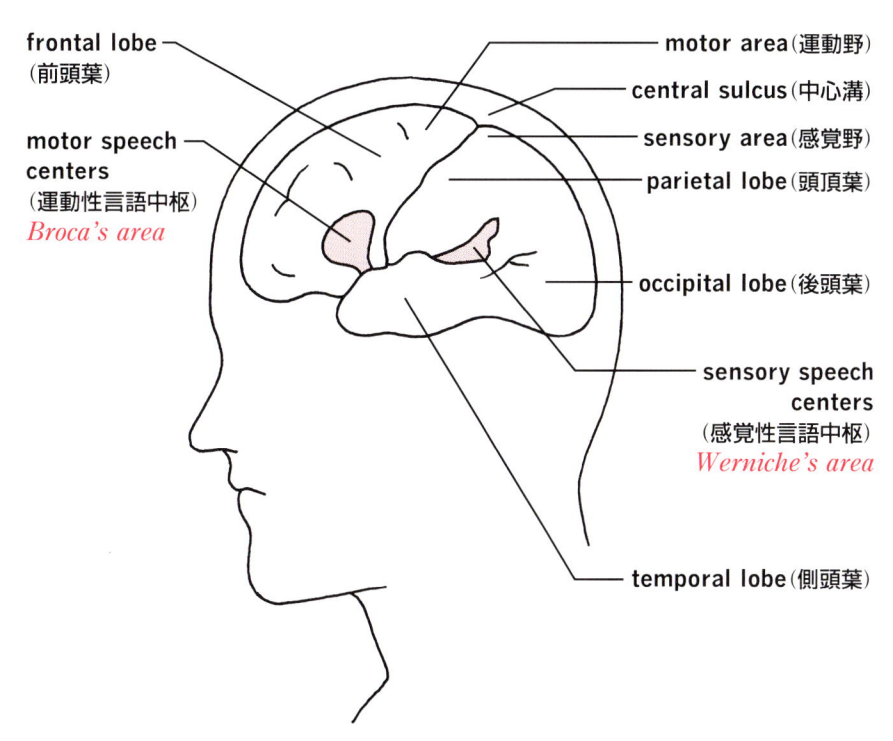

frontal lobe（前頭葉）
motor speech centers（運動性言語中枢）
Broca's area
motor area（運動野）
central sulcus（中心溝）
sensory area（感覚野）
parietal lobe（頭頂葉）
occipital lobe（後頭葉）
sensory speech centers（感覚性言語中枢）
Werniche's area
temporal lobe（側頭葉）

Fig 7-4　Speech centers（言語中枢）

Chapter 7

Questions 7(b)

Choose the best word from the list and fill in the blank.

1. When there is not enough blood going to part of the brain we get a _____.
2. The brain at the back part of head (occipital lobe) takes care of _____.
3. A patient with _____ may have difficulty with walking, eating, or other daily activities.
4. People with _____ disease do not have enough dopamine in their brain.
5. The first sign of Parkinson's disease is _____ of a limb.
6. _____ is one medicine that can help some people with Parkinson's disease.

| Parkinson's | paralysis | stroke | tremor | speaking |
| hearing | seeing | L-Dopa | | |

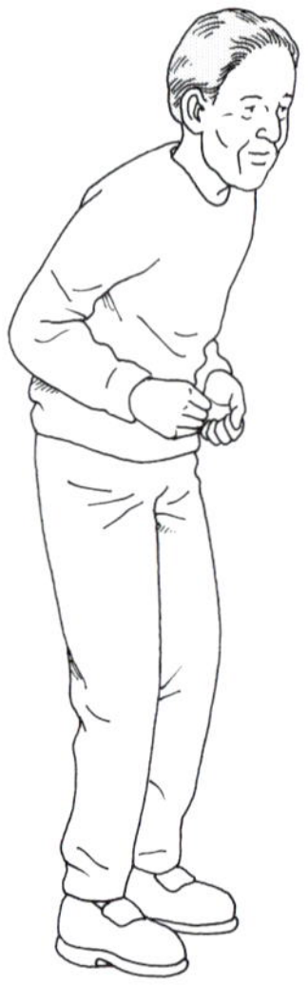

Fig 7-5　パーキンソン病の足を引きずる歩き方

Chapter 7

Vocabulary

cerebral edema	脳浮腫
cerebral hemorrhage	脳出血
intracerebral hemorrhage	脳内出血
extradural hemorrhage	硬膜外出血
subdural hemorrhage	硬膜下出血
subarachnoid hemorrhage (SAH)	クモ膜下出血
stroke	脳卒中
cerebral infarction	脳梗塞
cerebral thrombosis	脳血栓症
cerebral embolisim	脳塞栓症
cerebral palsy (CP)	脳性麻痺
quadriplegia (tetraplegia)	四肢麻痺
epilepsy	てんかん
partial seizure	部分発作
generalized seizure	全身性発作
Parkinson's disease (PD)	パーキンソン病
amytorophic lateral sclerosis (ALS)	筋萎縮性側索硬化症
multiple sclerosis (MS)	多発性硬化症
viral encephalitis	ウイルス性脳炎
AIDS encephalopathy	エイズ脳症
Creutzfeldt-Jakob disease (CJD)	クロイツフェルト・ヤコブ病
Reye syndrome	ライ症候群
phenylketonuria	フェニルケトン尿症
acute anterior poliomyelitis	急性灰白髄炎
peripheral neuropathies	末梢神経障害
trigeminal neuralgia	三叉神経痛
dementia	認知症
Alzheimer type dementia	アルツハイマー型認知症
cerebrovascular dementia	脳血管型認知症
schizophrenia	統合失調症

Chapter 7

manic-depressive psychosis	躁うつ病
mania	躁病
depression	うつ病
delirium	せん妄
amnesia	健忘
autism	自閉症
neurosis	ノイローゼ
anxiety neurosis	不安神経症
psychosomatic disorder	心身症

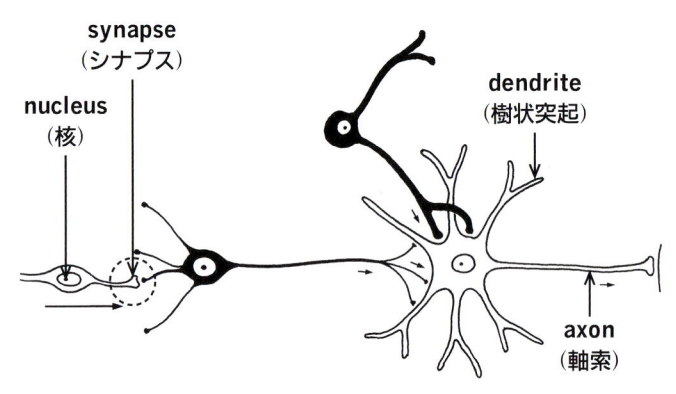

Fig 7-6 Linkage of neurons（ニューロンの連鎖）

接頭辞・接尾辞

接頭・接尾	意味	例
intra-	内(within)	intracerebral
extra-	外(outside)	extradural
sub-	下(under)	subarachinoid
-algia	～痛(pain)	neuralgia
-ia	～症(病気の状態)	schizophrenia, dementia, mania
-itis	～炎(炎症)	encephalitis
-osis	～症(疾病の過程・状況・状態)	thrombosis, psychosis, sclerosis
-pathy	～症，～療法	encephalopathy, neuropathy
-uria	～尿症(尿中に～の存在する状態)	phenylketonuria
-plegia	～麻痺	quadriplegia, tetraplegia

Chapter 7

神経系の語根

語根の連結形	意味
neur/o	神経(nerve)
gangli/o	神経節(ganglion)
cephal/o	頭(head)
encephal/o	脳(brain)
cerebr/o	大脳(cerebrum)
cerebell/o	小脳(cerebellum)
crani/o	頭蓋(skull)
mening/o, mening/i	髄膜(meninx)
myel/o	脊髄(spinal cord)　骨髄(marrow)
esthesi/o	感覚(sense)，知覚(perception)
narc/o	麻酔，昏睡
alge-, algesi/o, algio-, algo-	痛み(pain)
psych/o	精神(mind)
epilept/i, epilept/o	てんかん(epilepsy)

練習問題 7

1. -itis(〜炎)とつないで次の用語をつくりなさい。
    1　脳炎　_____　　2　脳脊髄炎　_____
    3　神経炎　_____　　4　(脳脊)髄膜炎　_____
    5　多発神経炎　_____

2. -oma(腫瘍)とつないで次の用語をつくりなさい。
    1　脳腫瘍　_____　　2　神経腫　_____
    3　神経節腫　_____　　4　髄膜腫　_____

3. -pathy(〜症，病気)とつないで次の用語をつくりなさい。
    1　神経障害　_____　　2　脳障害(脳症)　_____

Chapter 7

4. -plegia（麻痺）を含む次の用語の意味をいいなさい。

　　1　hemiplegia _____　　2　paraplegia _____
　　3　monoplegia _____　　4　diplegia _____
　　5　triplegia _____
　　6　tetraplegia (quadriplegia) _____

5. -esthesia（感覚，知覚）とつないで次の用語をつくりなさい。

　　1　感覚消失（触覚消失）_____　　2　感覚鈍麻（触覚鈍麻）_____
　　3　感覚過敏（触覚過敏）_____　　4　痛覚過敏 _____

6. 次の用語の意味をいいなさい。

　　1　anesthesia _____　　2　anesthesiology _____
　　3　anesthesiologist _____　　4　hemianesthesia _____
　　5　local anesthetic _____　　6　general anesthetic _____

7. psycho-（精神）を含む次の用語の意味をいいなさい。

　　1　psychosis _____　　2　psychosomatic _____
　　3　psychology _____　　4　psychoanalysis _____
　　5　psychiatry _____　　6　psychotropic drug _____

8. a-（無）を含む次の用語の意味をいいなさい。

　　1　aphasia _____　　2　acalculia _____
　　3　agraphia _____　　4　alexia _____
　　5　apraxia _____　　6　agnosia _____

Chapter 7

9．日本語の意味を調べなさい。

神経系の略語

ACh, Ach	acetylcholine	
Ad	adrenaline	
ALS	amyotrophic lateral sclerosis	
ANS	autonomic nervous system	
CJD	Creutzfeldt-Jakob disease	
CNS	central nervous system	
CP	cerebral palsy	
CSF	cerebrospinal fluid	
CVA	cerebrovascular accident	
CVD	cerebrovascular disorder	
DA	dopamine	
ECT	electroconvulsive therapy	
EEG	electroencephalography electroencephalogram	
KJ	knee jerk	
LP	lumbar puncture	
MS	multiple sclerosis	
PD	Parkinson's disease	
PNS	peripheral nervous system	
PR	plantar reflex	
PTSD	post-traumatic stress disorder	
SAH	subarachnoid hemorrhage	
TIA	transient ischemic attack	

Chapter 8

Musculoskeletal System
(筋骨格系)

Overview

The skeleton (bones) gives us shape, protects us and lets us move.　Adults have 206 bones.　The bones join together to make (form) joints.　The end of each bone is covered with a material called cartilage.　Each joint is covered by a special bag called a synovial membrane.　Inside of this membrane there is a special fluid, like oil, that lets the bones move together smoothly and easily.　It is called synovial fluid.

Our bones are attached to each other (held together) by strong bands (like rubber) which can stretch.　They are called ligaments.　Muscles are connected to bones by a special inelastic tissue called tendon.

Almost half the body's weight is muscle.　There are more than 640 muscles, and they hardly ever work alone.　Muscles get messages from nerves and they can get shorter (contract) and pull but they cannot push.　So, muscles are arranged in opposing teams.　One team pulls the body part one way, the other team relaxes and gets stretched.　Muscles band grip together to form muscle groups which work together.

skeleton（骨格）

joint（関節）
cartilage（軟骨）
synovial membrane（滑膜）
fluid（液体）

stretch（伸びる）
ligament（靱帯）
muscle（筋肉）
tendon（腱）

contract（収縮する）

relax（弛緩する）

Chapter 8

Voluntary muscles, such as your arms and legs can be controlled by your thoughts. The brain automatically controls involuntary muscles, such as the heart and breathing muscles. We don't have to think about making them work.

voluntary（随意の）
thought（思考）
involuntary（不随意の）

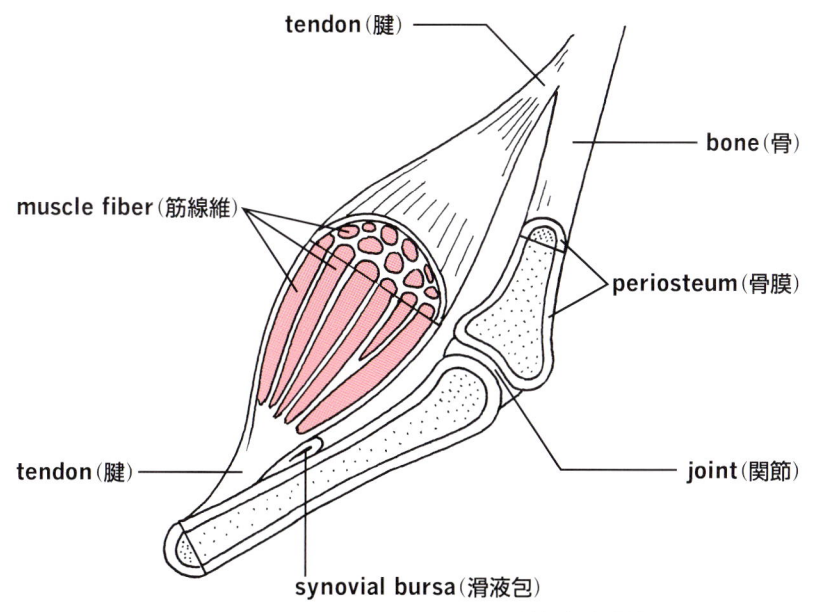

Fig 8-1　Muscle and bone（筋肉と骨）

Questions　8(a)

Choose the best word from the list and fill in the blank.

1. The skeleton (bones) gives us _____, protects us and lets us move.
2. The end of each bone is covered with a material called _____.
3. Our bones are attached to each other by strong bands called _____.
4. Joints are in a special bag called a _____ membrane.
5. Muscles are connected to bones by a special inelastic tissue called _____.
6. _____ muscles are controlled by your thoughts.
7. _____ muscles are automatically controlled by the brain.

ligaments	synovial	involuntary	smooth	shape
voluntary	skeletal	cartilage	tendon	

71

Chapter 8

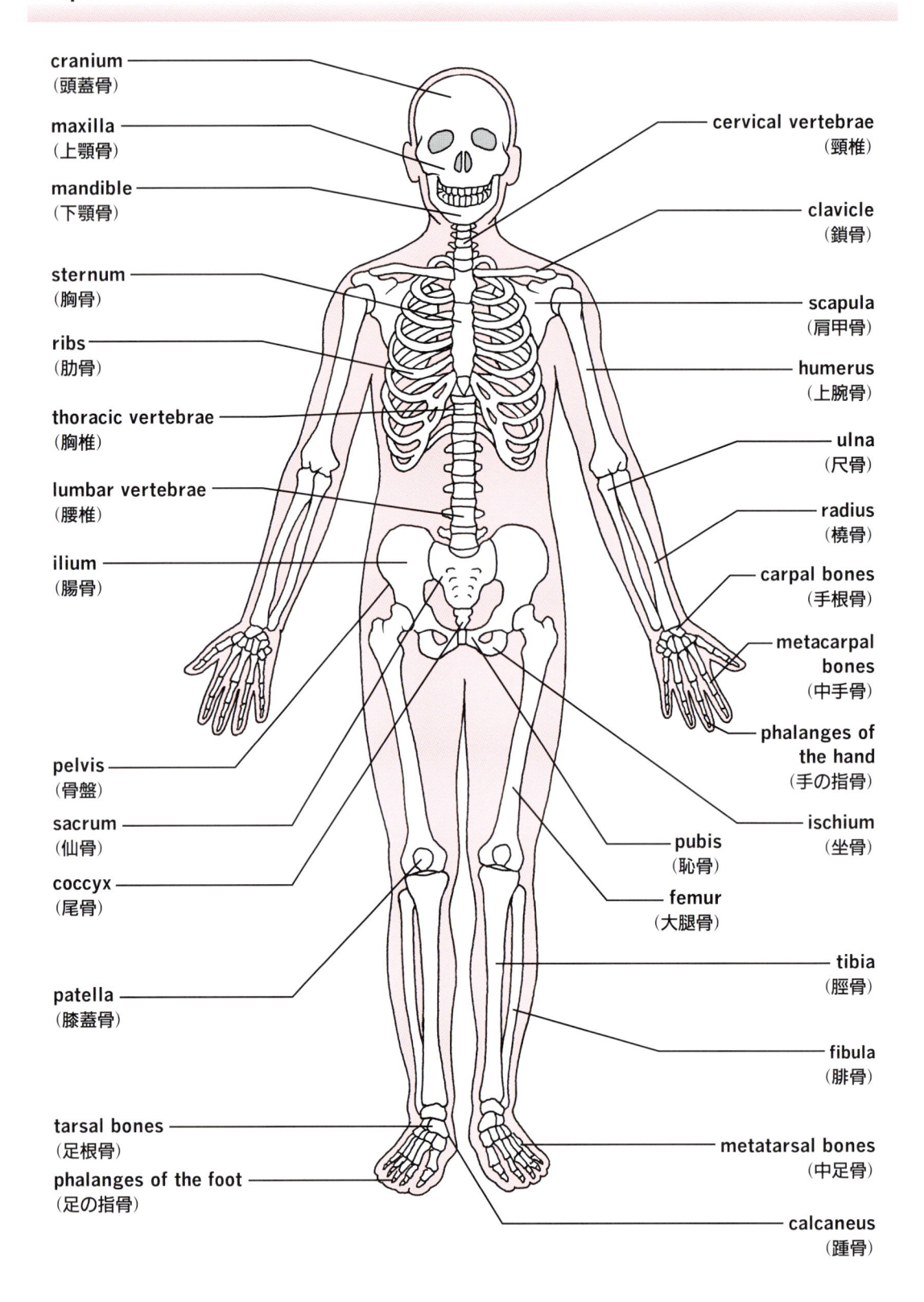

- cranium（頭蓋骨）
- maxilla（上顎骨）
- mandible（下顎骨）
- sternum（胸骨）
- ribs（肋骨）
- thoracic vertebrae（胸椎）
- lumbar vertebrae（腰椎）
- ilium（腸骨）
- pelvis（骨盤）
- sacrum（仙骨）
- coccyx（尾骨）
- patella（膝蓋骨）
- tarsal bones（足根骨）
- phalanges of the foot（足の指骨）
- cervical vertebrae（頸椎）
- clavicle（鎖骨）
- scapula（肩甲骨）
- humerus（上腕骨）
- ulna（尺骨）
- radius（橈骨）
- carpal bones（手根骨）
- metacarpal bones（中手骨）
- phalanges of the hand（手の指骨）
- ischium（坐骨）
- pubis（恥骨）
- femur（大腿骨）
- tibia（脛骨）
- fibula（腓骨）
- metatarsal bones（中足骨）
- calcaneus（踵骨）

Fig 8-2　Skeletal system（骨格系）

Chapter 8

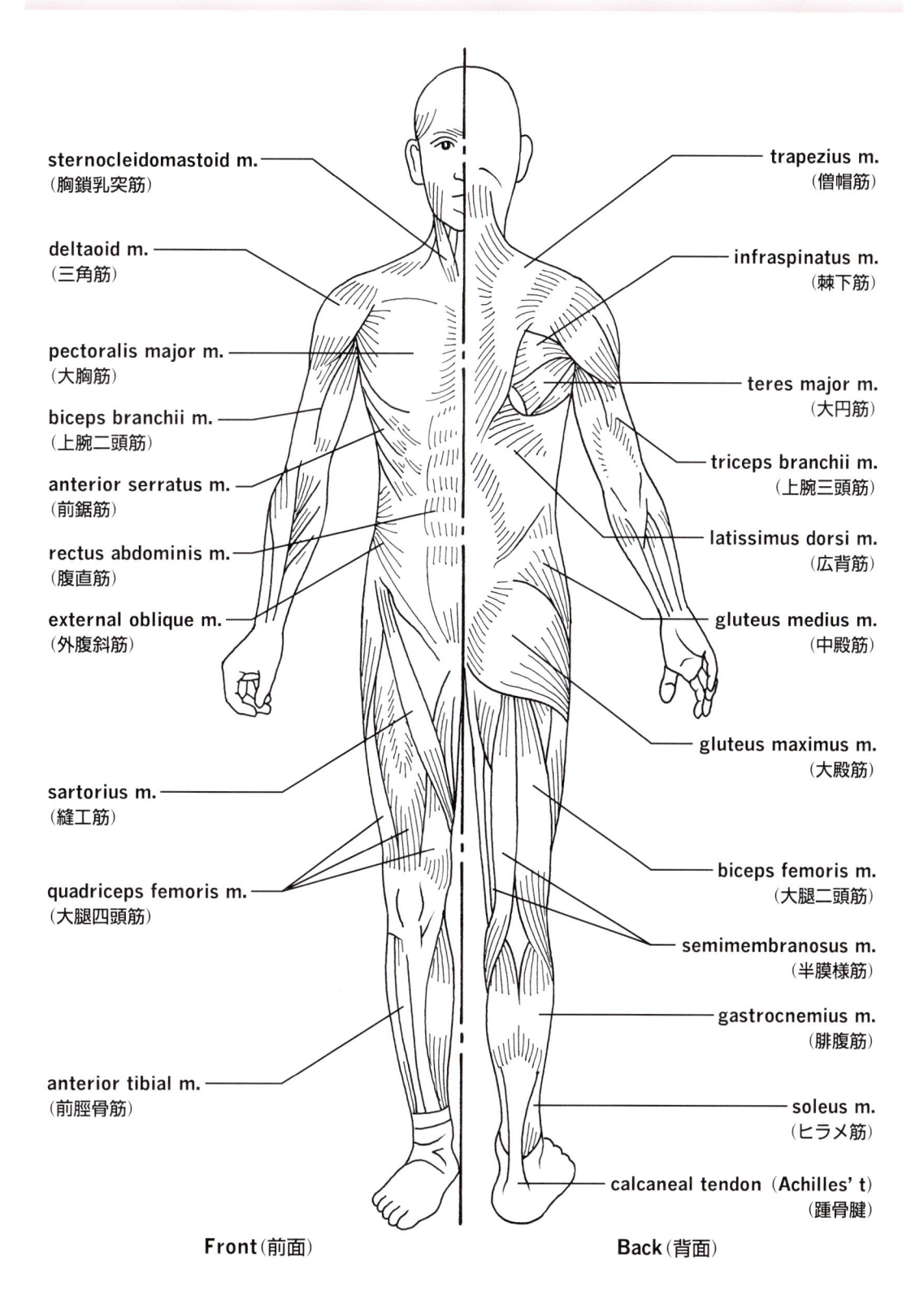

Front (前面)

- sternocleidomastoid m. (胸鎖乳突筋)
- deltaoid m. (三角筋)
- pectoralis major m. (大胸筋)
- biceps branchii m. (上腕二頭筋)
- anterior serratus m. (前鋸筋)
- rectus abdominis m. (腹直筋)
- external oblique m. (外腹斜筋)
- sartorius m. (縫工筋)
- quadriceps femoris m. (大腿四頭筋)
- anterior tibial m. (前脛骨筋)

Back (背面)

- trapezius m. (僧帽筋)
- infraspinatus m. (棘下筋)
- teres major m. (大円筋)
- triceps branchii m. (上腕三頭筋)
- latissimus dorsi m. (広背筋)
- gluteus medius m. (中殿筋)
- gluteus maximus m. (大殿筋)
- biceps femoris m. (大腿二頭筋)
- semimembranosus m. (半膜様筋)
- gastrocnemius m. (腓腹筋)
- soleus m. (ヒラメ筋)
- calcaneal tendon (Achilles' t) (踵骨腱)

Fig 8-3 Muscular system (筋肉系)

Chapter 8

Disorders of the Musculoskeletal System
(筋骨格系の疾患)

One common disease of the skeletal system is osteoporosis. The bones of the body become weak and fragile (easy to break). This is because the basic material of the bone, calcium (Ca), is going away. People with this problem can easily break or fracture bones, especially the hip, spine and wrist. The disease takes many years to show symptoms (signs) so it is often called the "silent disease".

Arthritis is a disease that occurs (is found) in the joints (*arthro* means joint). There are two main kinds: osteo and rheumatoid arthritis. Remember the word *osteo* means bone, so we can guess that osteoarthritis (OA) is a problem of the bone in the joint. This is the most common type of arthritis. The cartilage cushion in the joints breaks down. The bones rub together and there is pain and stiffness. Sometimes the rubbing makes new rough bones to grow. We call these bone growths, spurs.

Rheumatoid arthritis (RA) is when our immune system attacks the synovial tissue in the joint. This makes the joint inflamed (swelled up) and can change the shape of the joint area. Often, it is impossible to move or bend the joint.

Muscular dystrophy (MD) is a name we use for a group of

---

osteoporosis（骨粗鬆症）
fragile（もろい）
material（物質）

fracture（骨折する）
hip（腰）
spine（脊椎）
wrist（手首）
arthritis（関節炎）

rheumatoid arthritis（関節リウマチ）
osteoarthritis（変形性関節炎）

cartilage（軟骨）
stiffness（強直）
rubbing（摩擦）
spurs（棘，棘突起）

synovial tissue（滑膜組織）
inflame（炎症を起こす）

muscular dystrophy（筋ジストロフィー）

Chapter 8

muscle disorders (myopathies). It seems to come from our parents DNA. The muscles of the body slowly get weaker and weaker and may stop working. There are different types of muscular dystrophy. Though all types are rare the most common form is Duchenne MD. It is known that a gene defect (problems) is responsible for the onset of this disease.

myopathies(筋疾患)

rare(まれな)

gene defect(遺伝子の欠陥)

onset(始まり)

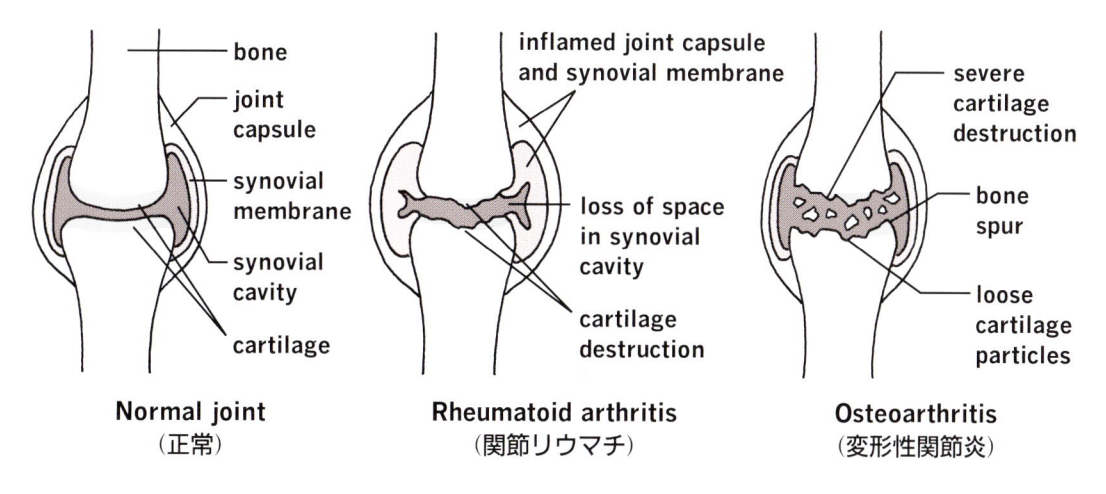

Normal joint (正常) — bone, joint capsule, synovial membrane, synovial cavity, cartilage

Rheumatoid arthritis (関節リウマチ) — inflamed joint capsule and synovial membrane, loss of space in synovial cavity, cartilage destruction

Osteoarthritis (変形性関節炎) — severe cartilage destruction, bone spur, loose cartilage particles

Fig 8-4 Arthritis(関節炎)

Questions 8(b)

Choose the best word from the list and fill in the blank.

1. The bones of the body become weak and fragile in _____, because calcium of the bone is going away.
2. Arthritis is a disease that occurs in the _____.
3. _____ is a problem of the bones in the joint.
4. _____ arthritis is when our immune system attacks the synovial tissue in the joint.
5. It is known that a gene defect is responsible for the onset of _____ muscular dystrophy.

rheumatoid	osteoarthritis	myopathies	osteoporosis
Duchenne	joints	spurs	

Chapter 8

Vocabulary

contracture	拘縮
quadriceps muscle contracture	大腿四頭筋拘縮
muscular atrophy (myoatrophy)	筋萎縮
disuse muscular atrophy	廃用性筋萎縮
progressive muscular dystrophy (PMD)	進行性筋ジストロフィー
myasthenia gravis	重症筋無力症
polymyositis	多発性筋炎
rhabdomyosarcoma	横紋筋肉腫
tendovaginitis	腱鞘炎
fracture	骨折
osteomalacia	骨軟化症
osteoporosis	骨粗鬆症
osteonecrosis	骨壊死
osteonecrosis of femoral head	大腿骨頭壊死
osteomyelitis	骨髄炎
osteochondroma	軟骨腫
osteosarcoma	骨肉腫
disuse bone atrophy	廃用性骨萎縮
dislocation	脱臼
sprain	捻挫
arthritis	関節炎
osteoarthritis (OA)	変形性関節炎
(degenerative arthritis)	
rheumatoid arthritis (RA)	関節リウマチ
gouty arthritis	通風性関節炎
arthralgia	関節痛
herniated intervertebral disc	椎間板ヘルニア
(prolapsed intervertebral disc, PID)	
lumbago (low back pain)	腰痛(症)

Chapter 8

接頭辞・接尾辞

接頭・接尾	意味	例
a-	無，不，非(not)	atrophy
dys-	変質，異常，悪い，困難	dystrophy
-algia	〜痛	arthralgia
-ia	〜症(異常な状態)	myasthenia, osteomalacia
-itis	〜炎(炎症)	arthritis, osteomyelitis, polyomyositis, tendovaginitis
-oma	腫瘍，新生物	osteochondroma, osteosarcoma, rhabdomyosarcoma
-osis	〜症(疾病の過程・状況・状態)	osteoporosis, osteonecrosis
-trophy	食物，栄養	atrophy, dystrophy

コラム 数量の用語

ギリシャ語系	ラテン語系	意味	
mon/o	uni-	1	(one, single)
di-, dipl/o	bi-	2	(two, double)
tri-, tripl/o	tri-	3	(three, triple)
tetr/a,	quadr/i, quart/i	4	(four, fourth)
pent/a	quinqu/e, quint/i	5	(five, fifth)
hex/a	sex/i, sext/i	6	(six, sixth)
hept/a	sept/i	7	(seven, seventh)
oct/i, oct/a	oct/i, oct/a	8	(eight, eighth)
non/a	non/i	9	(nine, ninth)
dec/a	dec/i	10	(ten, tenth)
pol/y	mult/i	多	(many)
hemi-	semi-	半分	(half)
olig/o		乏	(little)
	null/i	無	(none)

Chapter 8

筋骨格系の語根

語根の連結形	意味
my/o, myos/o, muscul/o	筋肉 (muscle)
lei/o leiomy/o	平滑 (smooth) 平滑筋 (smooth muscle)
rhabd/o rhabdomy/o	棒状 (rod) 横紋筋 (striated muscle)
sarc/o	肉 (flesh)
fasci/o	筋膜 (fascia)
aponeur/o	腱膜 (aponeurosis)
kin, kine, kinesi/o, kines/o, kinet/o	運動 (motion)
oste/o	骨 (bone)
calci/o	カルシウム (calcium)
rach/i, rachi/o, spondyl/o	脊椎, 脊柱 (spine)
disc/o	椎間板 (disc)
lamin/i, lamin/o	板 (plate)
myel/o	骨髄 (marrow)
cervic/i, cervic/o	くび, 頸部 (neck)
thorac/i, thrac/o	胸 (thorax)
lumb/o	腰椎 (loin)
arthr/o, articul/o	関節 (joint)
synovi/o	滑液 (synovial fluid)
burs/o	包, 嚢 (滑液の入った袋)
chondr/o	軟骨 (cartilage)
ten/o, tenont/o, tend/o, tendin/o	腱 (cord)
syndesm/o	靱帯 (ligament)
ankyl/o	屈曲 (bent)

Chapter 8

主な骨の語根

語根の連結形	意味
crani/o	頭蓋骨(cranium, skull)
maxill/o	上顎骨(maxilla)
submaxill/o, mandibul/o	下顎骨(submaxilla)
clavicul/o	鎖骨(clavicle)
scapul/o	肩甲骨(scapula)
cost/o	肋骨(rib)
stern/o	胸骨(sternum)
humer/o	上腕骨(humerus)
uln/o	尺骨(ulna)
olecran/o	肘(olecranon)
radi/o	橈骨(radius)
carp/o	手根，手首の骨(carpus)
metacarp/o	中手骨(手骨)(metacarpus)
phalang/o	指節骨(phalanx)
pelv/i	骨盤(pelvis)
ill/o	腸骨(illium)
ischi/o	坐骨(ischium)
pub/o	恥骨(pubis)
acetabul/o	寛骨臼(acetabulus)
femor/o	大腿骨(femur)
patell/o	膝蓋骨(patella)
tibi/o	脛骨(tibia)
fibul/o, perone/o	腓骨(fibular)
calcane/o	踵骨(calcaneus)

Chapter 8

練習問題 8

1. -itis（〜炎）とつないで次の用語をつくりなさい。
    1　筋炎　_____　2　骨炎　_____
    3　関節炎　_____　4　腱鞘炎　_____

2. -oma（腫，腫瘍）とつないで次の用語をつくりなさい。
    1　筋腫　_____　2　平滑筋腫　_____
    3　横紋筋腫　_____　4　骨腫　_____
    5　軟骨腫　_____　6　骨髄腫　_____

3. -sarcoma（肉腫）とつないで次の用語をつくりなさい。
    1　筋肉腫　_____　2　骨肉腫　_____

4. -plasty（形成術）とつないで次の用語をつくりなさい。
    1　骨形成術　_____　2　軟骨形成術　_____
    3　関節形成術　_____　4　靱帯形成術　_____

5. -ectomy（切除術）とつないで次の用語をつくりなさい。
    1　骨切除術　_____　2　軟骨切除術　_____
    3　関節切除術　_____

6. -dystrophy（異栄養症，栄養失調症）とつないで次の用語をつくりなさい。
    1　筋ジストロフィー　_____　2　骨ジストロフィー　_____

7. -dysplasia（形成異常症，異形成症）とつないで次の用語をつくりなさい。
    1　軟骨形成不全症（軟骨異形成症）　_____
    2　関節形成不全症　_____

8. -malacia（軟化症）とつないで次の用語をつくりなさい。
    1　骨軟化症　_____　2　軟骨軟化症　_____

Chapter 8

9．次の用語の意味をいいなさい。

1　myalgia　＿＿＿＿＿＿＿＿＿＿　2　myasthenia　＿＿＿＿＿＿＿＿＿＿
3　synovitis　＿＿＿＿＿＿＿＿＿＿　4　osteoblast　＿＿＿＿＿＿＿＿＿＿
5　osteoclast　＿＿＿＿＿＿＿＿＿＿　6　osteoporosis　＿＿＿＿＿＿＿＿＿＿

10．日本語の意味を調べなさい。

筋・骨格系の略語

BI	bone injury	
C1, C2, etc	cervical vertebrae	
CDH	congenital dislocation of hip joint	
DTR	deep tendon reflex	
EMG	electromyogram/electromyography	
Fx	fracture	
L1, L2, etc	lumbar vertebrae	
MAP	muscle action potential	
MFT	muscle function test	
MNJ	myoneural junction	
OA	osteoarthritis	
Ortho	orthopedics	
PID	prolapsed intervertebral disc	
PMD	progressive muscular dystrophy	
RA	rheumatoid arthritis	
RF (Rhf)	rheumatoid factor	
T1, T2, etc	thoracic vertebrae	
THR	total hip replacement	
TJ	triceps jerk	

Chapter 9

Skin and Sensory System
（皮膚および感覚器）

Overview

The body is connected to the outside world by the five senses. All living things have some way to feel the energy of the environment. A network of nerves in the skin gives us the most basic sense called touch. These different nerve endings gather information and send it to the brain. We call these feelings pressure, temperature and pain. This network of nerves making up touch is the largest sense organ. The next level of feeling the outside world is chemical. The nose and tongue detect smell and taste, respectively.

The tongue is covered with dozens of little bumps called papillae. These grip and move food when you chew. Around the sides of the papillae are (exist) about 10,000 microscopic taste buds. Different parts of the tongue are sensitive to different flavors: sweet, salt, sour and bitter.

Inside each side of the nose is an air chamber, called the nasal cavity. When we sniff, air swirls up into the top of the cavity. Here is a small patch of about 10 million specialized olfactory (smelling) cells. They have long micro-hairs, called cilia, sticking out from them. Odor particles in the air stick on the

touch（触覚）

detect（検出する）

bump（出っ張り）
papillae
（papilla, 乳頭の複数形）
microscopic（顕微鏡によらなければ見えない）
flavor（味わい）
chamber（部屋）
nasal cavity（鼻腔）
sniff（匂いをかぐ）
swirl（渦を巻く）
patch（断片）
olfactory cells
（嗅覚細胞）
cilia（cilium, 線毛の複数形）

Chapter 9

cilia and make the olfactory cells produce nerve signals. These signals travel to the olfactory bulb which is the first step in smelling. They continue along the olfactory tract to the brain where they are recognized as smells.

bulb(球)

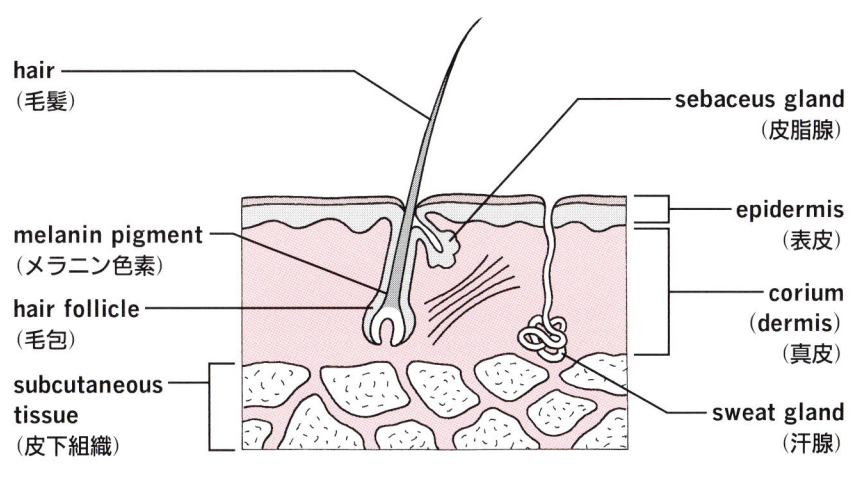

Fig 9-1　Skin（皮膚）

- hair（毛髪）
- sebaceus gland（皮脂腺）
- melanin pigment（メラニン色素）
- epidermis（表皮）
- hair follicle（毛包）
- corium（dermis）（真皮）
- subcutaneous tissue（皮下組織）
- sweat gland（汗腺）

Sound waves enter the ear and go down a narrow tube called the external ear canal. At the end is a small patch of rubbery skin known as the tympanic membrane (eardrum). The sound waves bounce off the tympanic membrane and make it shake (vibrate). The membrane is connected to a row of three tiny bones. They are linked together and are called the hammer, anvil and stirrup. The vibrations pass along these bones. The stirrup presses against the cochlea, deep inside the ear. The cochlea is small and shaped like a snail and is filled with fluid. The vibrations from the stirrup make the fluid ripple inside the cochlea.

external ear canal（外耳道）
rubbery（ゴムのような）
tympanic membrane（鼓膜）
bounce off（はずませる）
vibrate（振動する）
hammer（＝malleus，ツチ骨）
anvil（＝incus，キヌタ骨）
stirrup（＝stapes，アブミ）
cochlea（蝸牛）
snail（カタツムリ）
ripple（さざ波が立つ）

Chapter 9

Here, they shake thousands of tiny hairs in the fluid that are connected to hair cells. As the hairs shake, the hair cells make nerve signals, which go along the auditory nerve to the hearing center of the brain.

auditory nerve(聴覚神経)

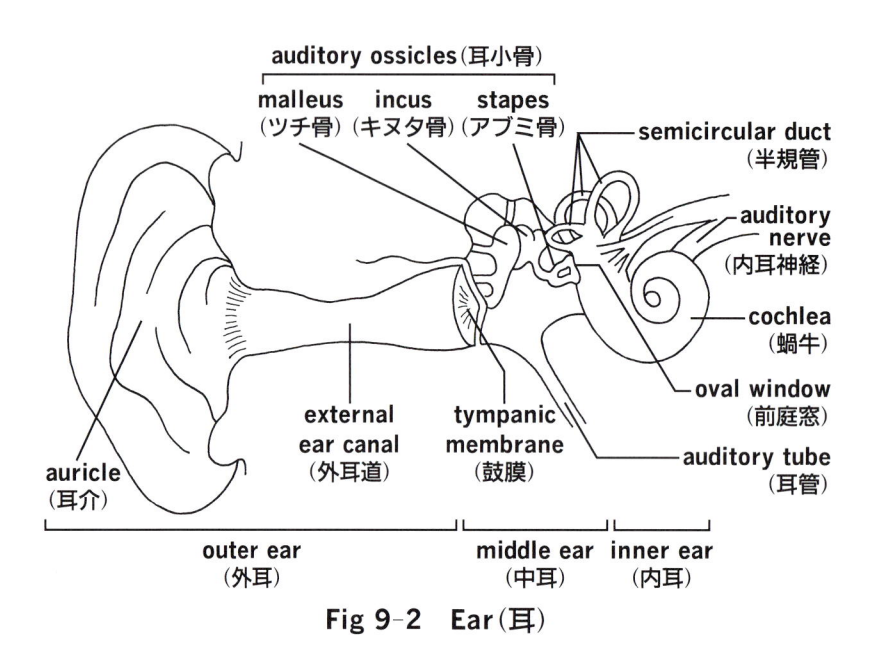

Fig 9-2　Ear(耳)

The most complicated of our senses is vision. The tough, white outer layer of the eyeball is called the sclera. Inside, there is a soft, blood-rich, nourishing layer, called the choroids. On the inner side of the choroid, around the sides and back of the eye, is the retina. The retina has special light receivers (receptors) called rods and cones. These receptors change light energy into chemical energy and then into nerve signals. These signals travel along the optic nerve to the brain. The eyeball is filled with a clear jelly called vitreous humor. At the front of the eye is the dome-shaped cornea, which lets the light in.

vision(視覚)
tough(強靱な)
eyeball(眼球)
sclera(強膜)
choroids(脈絡膜)
retina(網膜)
rod(かん体)
cone(錐体)
vitreous humor(硝子体液)
cornea(角膜)

Chapter 9

The light rays pass through a hole, the pupil, in a ring of muscle, called the iris. Then, the rays shine through the convex lens, which bends and focuses them to form a clear picture on the retina.

pupil（瞳孔）

iris（虹彩）

ray（光線）

convex lens（凸面レンズ）

lens（水晶体）

focus（焦点に集める）

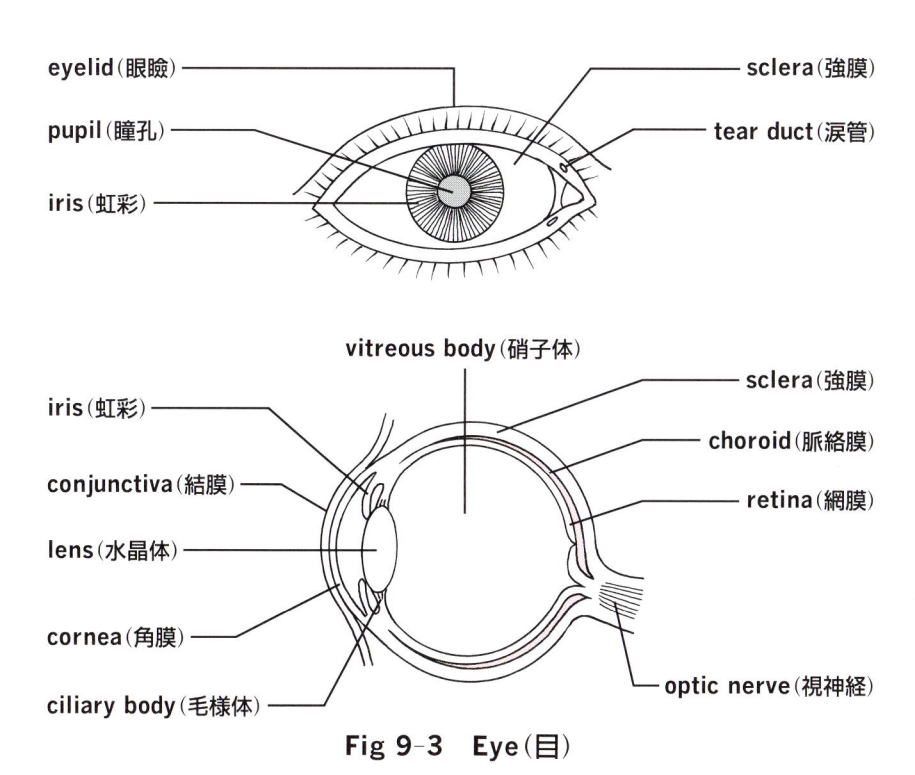

- eyelid（眼瞼）
- pupil（瞳孔）
- iris（虹彩）
- sclera（強膜）
- tear duct（涙管）

- iris（虹彩）
- conjunctiva（結膜）
- lens（水晶体）
- cornea（角膜）
- ciliary body（毛様体）
- vitreous body（硝子体）
- sclera（強膜）
- choroid（脈絡膜）
- retina（網膜）
- optic nerve（視神経）

Fig 9-3　Eye（目）

Chapter 9

Questions 9(a)

Choose the best word from the list and fill in the blank.

1. A network of nerves in the skin gives us the most basic sense called _____.
2. The tongue is covered with dozens of little bumps called _____.
3. Odor particles in the air stick on the cilia and make the _____ cells produce nerve signals.
4. The sound waves bounce off the _____ and make it shake (vibrate).
5. The tympanic membrane is connected to a row of three tiny bones linked together called hammer, _____ and stirrup.
6. The stirrup presses against the _____ which is small and shaped like a snail and is filled with fluid.
7. The _____ has special light receivers (receptors) called rods and cones.
8. At the front of the eye is the dome-shaped _____, through which light rays enter.
9. Light rays pass through a hole, called the _____, in a ring of muscle, called the _____.
10. The light rays shine through the convex _____, which bends and focuses them to form a clear picture on the retina.

cochlea	lens	pupil	anvil	touch	cornea
conjunctiva	retina	sclera	iris	papillae	choroids
tympanic membrane		olfactory			

Chapter 9

Disorders of the Skin and the Sensory System
(皮膚および感覚器系の疾患)

Skin

Atopic dermatitis or eczema is most common in infants but can occur at any age. It is an itchy, dry, hypersensitive skin disorder, but it is not infectious. No one knows the real cause of atopic dermatitis. Doctors do know that it has a genetic component. The patient or some family members may have other hypersensitive conditions such as asthma or hay fever.

atopic dermatitis (アトピー性皮膚炎)	
eczema (湿疹)	
itchy (かゆい)	
infectious (感染性の)	
component (成分)	
asthma (喘息)	
hay fever (枯草熱)	

Pressure sores or bedsores (also known as decubitus ulcer) are another common skin problem with people in hospitals or in wheelchairs. The skin is often painful, red and ulcerated. This is caused by pressure and lack of movement. The constant pressure against the skin causes decreased blood supply to that area and causes death (necrosis) of the affected tissue. The most common places for pressure ulcers are over bones close to the skin, such as the elbow, heel, hip, ankle, shoulder, back, and the back of the head. Moving the patient frequently, changing bedding, and keeping the skin clean and dry can prevent them.

pressure sore (床ずれ)
bedsore (床ずれ)
decubitus ulcer (褥瘡)
ulcerate (潰瘍をおこす)

ulcer (潰瘍)

Chapter 9

Ears

Motion sickness is a common disturbance of the inner ear (labyrinth). People can become motion sick in cars, airplanes, amusement park rides, boats or ships. Motion sickness is connected to the sense of balance and equilibrium. The symptoms of motion sickness include nausea, vomiting, and dizziness (vertigo). Other common signs are sweating and a general feeling of discomfort (malaise). Antihistamine medications are commonly used in the prevention and treatment of motion sickness.

Hearing loss, or deafness, can be present at birth (congenital) or later in life (acquired). Some congenital deafness may be due to infection which the mother had during pregnancy, such as the rubella virus. As you age, your hearing may decline, especially that of high-frequency sounds. This age-related hearing loss (presbycusis) is one of the most common acquired hearing problem in adults.

There are two types of hearing loss: *conductive or sensorineural*. *Conductive hearing loss* results from abnormality of the external ear and/or the ossicles of the middle ear. *Sensorineural hearing loss* occurs when inner ear structures (cochlea), or the auditory nerve or the brain, are damaged in some way.

---

motion sickness (動揺病，乗り物酔い)
malaise (倦怠感)
disturbance (障害)
labyrinth (内耳)
nausea (悪心，吐き気)
vomiting (嘔吐)
dizziness (めまい)
vertigo (めまい，眩そう)
discomfort (不快)
malaise (倦怠，不快)
antihistamine (抗ヒスタミン薬)
medication (薬物療法)
congenital (先天性)
acquired (後天性の)
pregnancy (妊娠)
rubella virus (風疹ウイルス)
high-frequency sound (高音)
presbycusis (老人性難聴)
hearing loss (難聴)
deafness (難聴)
conductive hearing loss (伝音性難聴)
ossicle (小骨)
sensorineural hearing loss (感音性難聴)
cochlea (蝸牛)
auditory nerve (聴覚神経)

Chapter 9

Eyes

Glaucoma is the main cause of irreversible blindness. Six million people worldwide are blind in both eyes from this disease. The eye is firm and round, like a basketball. Pressure within the eye (the intraocular pressure, IOP) maintains its tone and shape. This pressure is usually between 8 and 22 mm (millimeters) of mercury. When the pressure is too low, the eye becomes softer and if it is too high, the eye becomes harder. The optic nerve at the rear of the eye is very sensitive to intraocular high pressure. The delicate fibers in this nerve are easily damaged and cannot be repaired. Glaucoma takes a long time to show any signs (symptoms). People gradually (slowly) lose their peripheral (outer edge) vision first. If glaucoma is discovered early on, we can control the pressure by eye drops, laser, or surgery.

Cataract is another eye disease that comes with getting old. This disorder affects 60% of people older than 60. Cataract is a clouding of the lens portion of the eye. It is like smearing grease over the lens of a camera. The image (vision) will not be clear or normal. Today, the clouded lens is surgically removed and replaced with a plastic intraocular lens (IOL). The operation takes only an hour and often requires no hospitalization. Implantation of the lens is one of the most successful operations in medicine.

glaucoma（緑内障）

intraocular pressure（眼内圧）

optic nerve（視神経）
rear（後ろ）

symptom（症状）

eye drop（点眼剤）
laser（レーザー）

cataract（白内障）

lens（水晶体）
smear（塗りつける）
grease（グリース）
image（像）
vision（視覚）
hospitalization（入院）
implantation（移植）

Chapter 9

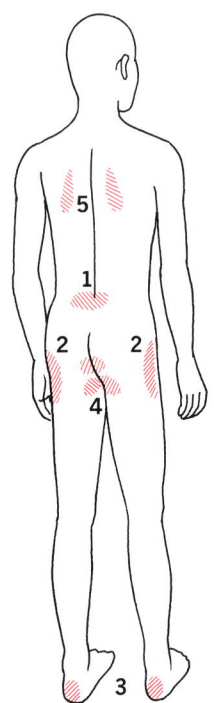

Fig 9-4　褥瘡の好発部位

1. 仙骨　　　　sacrum
2. 大転子　　　trochanter major
3. 踵骨　　　　calcaneus
4. 坐骨結節　　tuber ischiadicum
5. 肩甲骨　　　scapula

Questions 9(b)

Choose the best word from the list and fill in the blank.

1. An itchy, dry, hypersensitive skin disorder is _____.
2. Moving a patient frequently, changing bedding and keeping the skin clean and dry can prevent _____.
3. A very common disturbance of the inner ear is _____.
4. The symptoms of motion sickness include nausea, vomiting, and _____.
5. The main cause of irreversible blindness is _____.
6. A _____ clouds the lens portion of the eye.

bedsores	cataract	motion sickness	glaucoma
atopic dermatitis		dizziness	deafness

Chapter 9

Vocabulary

alopecia	脱毛(症)
acne	ざそう(にきび)
burns	熱傷，火傷
eruption	発疹
eczema	湿疹
keratosis	角化症
atopic dermatitis	アトピー性皮膚炎
contact dermatitis	接触性皮膚炎
herpes zoster	帯状疱疹
psoriasis	乾癬
pressure sores (decubitus ulcers)	床ずれ(褥瘡)
squamous cell carcinoma	扁平上皮癌
malignant melanoma	悪性黒色腫
stye (hordeolum)	麦粒腫(ものもらい)
blepharitis	眼瞼炎
conjunctivitis	結膜炎
trachoma	トラコーマ
uveitis	ぶどう膜炎
glaucoma	緑内障
cataract	白内障
diabetic retinopathy	糖尿病性網膜症
retinodialysis (retinal detachment)	網膜剝離
retinoblastoma	網膜芽細胞腫
retrolental fibroplasia	後水晶体線維増殖症(未熟児網膜症)
otitis externa	外耳炎
otitis media	中耳炎
otitis interna	内耳炎
Meniere's disease	メニエール病
motion sickness	乗り物酔い
sensorineural hearing impairment	感音性難聴
conductive hearing impairment	伝音性難聴

Chapter 9

allergic rhinitis	アレルギー性鼻炎
sinusitis	副鼻腔炎
trachyphonia (hoarseness)	嗄声(させい)
keratoplasty (transplantation of the cornea)	角膜移植(術)
emmetropia	正常視
hypermetropia	遠視
myopia	近視

接尾辞

接尾辞	意味	例
-itis	～炎(炎症)	dermatitis, blepharitis, conjunctivitis, uveitis, otitis, rhinitis, sinusitis
-ia	～症(病気の状態)	tachyphonia
-osis	～症(病的状態)	keratosis
-oma	腫瘍，新生物	melanoma, carcinoma, retinoblastoma
-pathy	病気	retinopathy
-plasia	形成，成長，発達	fibroplasia
-plasty	形成術(外科的手段による形成)	keratoplasty
-opia	視覚	hypermetropia, myopia, emmetropia

皮膚および感覚器の語根

語根の連結形	意味
derm/a, dermat/o, -derma	皮膚(skin)
kerat/o	角質(keratin)，角膜(cornea)
pil/o	毛(hair)
trich/o	毛髪(hair)
seb/o	皮脂(sebum)

Chapter 9

語根の連結形	意味
hidr/o	汗，汗腺(sweat)
onych/o	爪(nail)
melan/o	黒(black)
ophthalm/o, ocul/o, opt/o, optic/o	眼(eye)
cor/e, core/o, pupil/o	瞳孔(pupil)
corne/o, kerat/o	角膜(cornea)
scler/o	硬化(hard)，強膜(sclera)
ir/o, irid/o	虹彩(iris)
retin/o	網膜(retina)
cycl/o	毛様体(ciliary body)
uve/o	ぶどう膜(uvea)
dacry/o, lacrim/o	涙(tear)，涙嚢(tear sac)
conjunctiv/o	結膜(conjunctiva)
blephar/o	眼瞼(eyelid)
ot/o, aur/i	耳(ear)
myring/o	鼓膜(eardrum)
audi/o	聴覚(auditory, hearing)
rhin/o, nas/o	鼻(nose)
gloss/o	舌(tongue)

練習問題 9

1. -itis（～炎）とつないで次の用語をつくりなさい。

    1 皮膚炎 _____   2 角膜炎 _____
    3 眼瞼炎 _____   4 結膜炎 _____
    5 ぶどう膜炎 _____   6 耳炎 _____
    7 鼻炎 _____   8 舌炎 _____

2. -plasty（形成術）とつないで次の用語をつくりなさい。

    1 角膜形成術(移植)_____   2 鼓膜形成術_____

Chapter 9

3. -ist（～する人）を含む次の用語の意味をいいなさい。

　　1　oculist _____　　2　ophthalmologist _____
　　3　dermatologist _____　　4　otolaryngologist _____

4. opto-（眼）を含む次の用語の意味をいいなさい。

　　1　optometer _____　　2　optometry _____
　　3　optometrist _____　　4　optomyometer _____

5. -opia（視覚）を含む次の用語の意味をいいなさい。

　　1　diplopia _____　　2　presbyopia _____
　　3　amblyopia _____　　4　achromatopsia _____

6. audio-（聴覚）を含む次の用語の意味をいいなさい。

　　1　audiology _____　　2　audiometer _____
　　3　audiogram _____　　4　audiometry _____

7. -scope（～鏡），-scopy（見る術，検査）を含む次の用語の意味をいいなさい。

　　1　auriscope _____　　2　auriscopy _____
　　3　otoscope _____　　4　otoscopy _____

8. 次の用語の意味をいいなさい。

　　1　keratosis _____　　2　keratolysis _____
　　3　retinodialysis _____　　4　retinoblastoma _____
　　5　blepharoptosis _____　　6　blepharoedema _____
　　7　rhinorrhagia _____　　8　rhinophonia _____
　　9　dysphonia _____　　10　aphonia _____

Chapter 9

9. 日本語の意味を調べなさい。
皮膚および感覚器の略語

bx	biopsy	
Derm	dermatology	
LA	local anesthetic	
ST	skin test	
Subcu.	subcutaneous	
ung	ointment	
OD	oculus dexter (right eye)	
OS	oculus sinister (left eye)	
Ophth	ophtha	
VA	visual acuity	
VF	visual field	
AD	auris dextra (right ear)	
AS	auris sinistra (left ear)	
aud	audiology	
ENT	ear nose and throat	
OE	otitis externa	
OM	otitis media	
oto	otology	
NAS	nasal	
NP	nasopharynx	

Chapter 10

Reproductive System
(生殖器系)

Overview

The human reproductive system is different from the other systems because it has male and female parts (sexual components). The word sexual means animals or plants that need two different members to make a baby (offspring). The female makes a large cell for reproduction called an ovum (egg). The male makes a smaller reproductive cell called a spermatozoon (sperm).

In the male reproductive system sperm are produced in the testes, which are contained in the scrotum, an external sac in the groin. The testes also produce the male hormone, testosterone. They also make some of the liquid in which sperm are carried. The scrotum is about 2°C cooler than the rest of the body and this condition is important for sperm development. After sperm are made, they pass from the testes into other important parts of the system. These parts produce (make) nutrients and an alkaline fluid in which sperm live. Sperm and the fluid (called semen) are finally carried to the ejaculatory duct (pipe). This duct is connected to the urethra. Sperm pass through the urethra from the man into the woman during intercourse.

components	(成分，構成要素)
offspring	(子，子孫)
reproduction	(生殖)
spermatozoon	(＝sperm 精子)
testes	(精巣，testis の複数形)
scrotum	(陰嚢)
sac	(嚢)
groin	(鼠けい)
semen	(精液)
ejaculatory duct	(射精管)
urethra	(尿道)
intercourse	(性交)

Chapter 10

In the human female reproductive system, ova (eggs) are made (produced) in the ovaries. The ovaries consist of two small organs on each side of the lower abdomen. The ovaries secrete (release) the hormones, estrogen and progesterone. Usually, each month an egg is released from one ovary and it passes into the fallopian (uterine) tube. If sperm are present, fertilization occurs within the tube. The ovum, either fertilized or unfertilized, goes down the fallopian tube and into the womb (uterus). The uterus is a pear-shaped organ which can feed and protect the fertilized egg. The egg grows into an embryo, fetus, and finally an infant. Approximately 10 months after fertilization the new baby is born and passes out through the vagina (birth canal). Sometimes, for medical reasons, the baby is removed surgically by cesarean section.

ova（卵・卵子，ovum の複数形）
ovaries（卵巣，ovary の複数形）
abdomen（腹）
secrete（分泌する）
release（放出する）
fallopian tube（ファロピウス管）
uterine tube（卵管）
fertilization（受精）
womb（＝uterus 子宮）
embryo（胚，胎児）
fetus（胎児）
infant（乳児）
vagina（膣）
cesarean section（帝王切開）

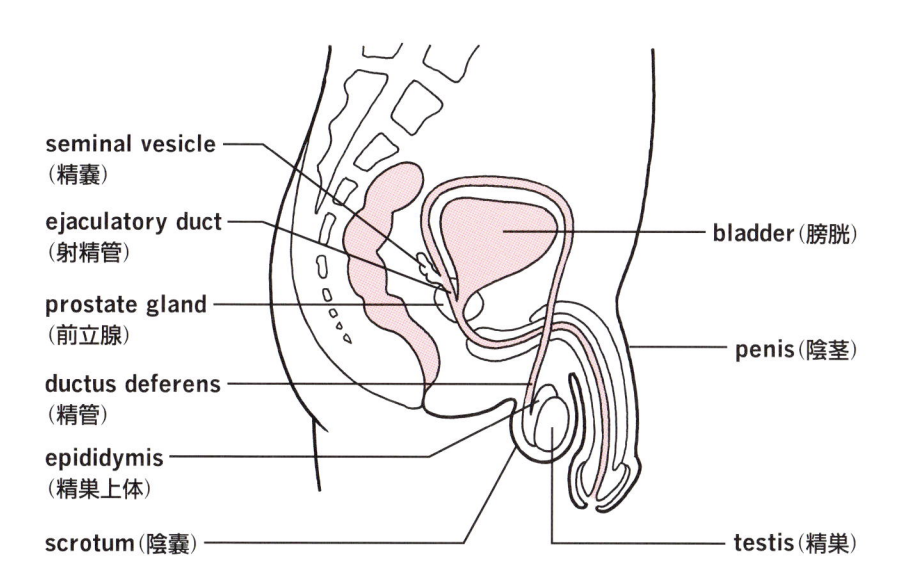

Fig 10-1　Male reproductive system（男性生殖器）

- seminal vesicle（精嚢）
- ejaculatory duct（射精管）
- prostate gland（前立腺）
- ductus deferens（精管）
- epididymis（精巣上体）
- scrotum（陰嚢）
- bladder（膀胱）
- penis（陰茎）
- testis（精巣）

Chapter 10

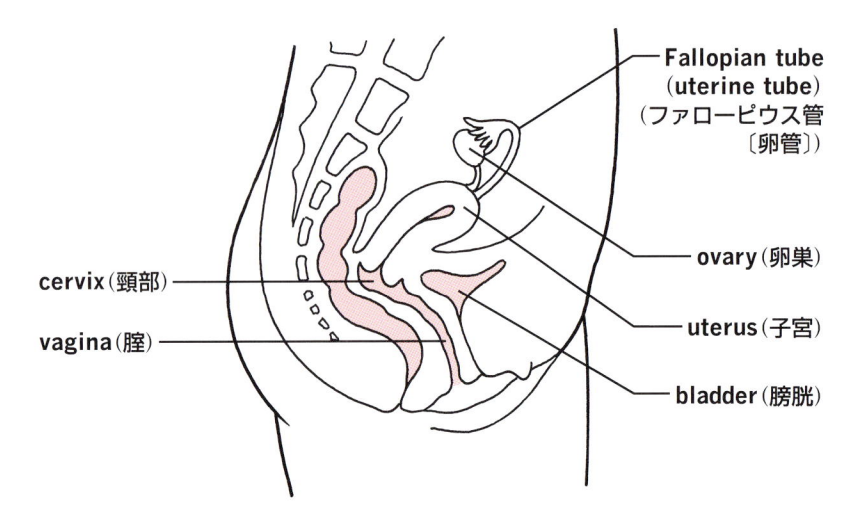

Fig 10-2 Female reproductive system(女性生殖器)

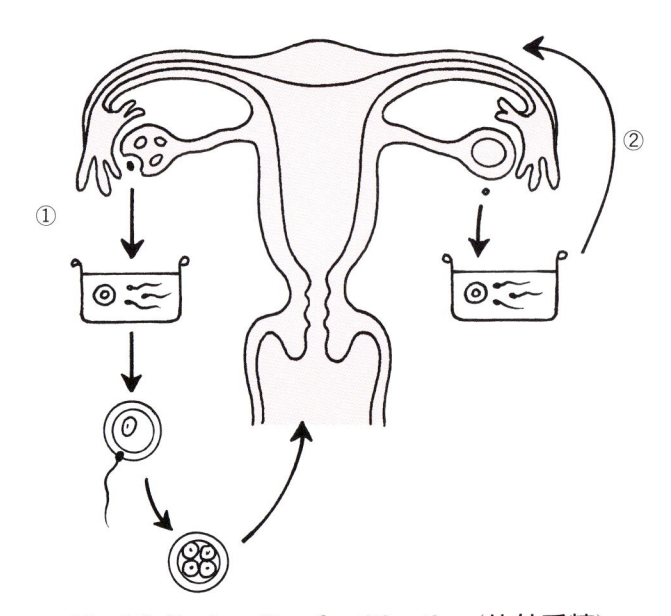

- Fallopian tube (uterine tube)（ファロービウス管〔卵管〕）
- ovary（卵巣）
- uterus（子宮）
- bladder（膀胱）
- cervix（頸部）
- vagina（腟）

Fig 10-3 In vitro fertilization(体外受精)
①IVF-ET 法（胚を子宮内に戻す）
　IVF-ET: in vitro fertilization and embryo transfer
②GIFT 法（培養せずに卵管内に戻す）
　GIFT: gamete-intra fallopian transfer（卵管内配偶子移植法）

Chapter 10

Questions 10(a)

Choose the best word from the list and fill in the blank.

1. The large reproductive cell made by females is a(n) _____.
2. The ovaries secrete the hormones, _____ and progesterone.
3. The ovum goes down the _____ tube and into the womb (uterus).
4. The _____ is a pear-shaped organ which feeds and protects the fertilized egg.
5. Sperm are produced in the _____.
6. The external sac in the groin of the male is called _____.
7. The testes also produce the male hormone _____.
8. The semen are carried to the _____ duct.

ejaculatory	ovum	fallopian	vagina	uterus
testosterone	scrotum	epididymis	testes	estrogen

コラム

色に関する用語（連結形）

連結形	意味	例
chrom/o, chromat/o	色 (color)	chromatin（染色質）
leuk/o, leuc/o	白 (white)	leukocyte（白血球）
melan/o	黒 (black)	melanoma（黒色腫）
erythr/o	赤 (red)	erythrocyte（赤血球）
cyan/o	青 (blue)	cyanosis（チアノーゼ）
chlor/o	緑 (green)	chloroplast（葉緑体）
xanth/o	黄 (yellow)	xanthoma（黄色腫）
glauk/o, glauc/o	灰緑 (bluish green)	glaucoma（緑内障）

Chapter 10

Disorders of the Reproductive System
（生殖器系の疾患）

We have seen that the male and female reproductive systems are quite different. However, disorders can occur in both men and women because of abnormal hormone secretion, sexually transmitted diseases (STD) or tumor growth.

Infertility occurs when the man's sperm can not fertilize the woman's egg (conceive/conception) or when the embryo or fetus cannot finish development and be delivered. The term *sterility* means that a man cannot make sperm or a woman cannot ovulate (release eggs from the ovary). Many factors can cause infertility in a woman. The egg may not come out of the ovary properly or it may not move down the fallopian tube. Even if the egg is fertilized by the sperm, it might not implant to the inside of the uterus. New technology such as IVF and GIFT can solve many of these problems.

As men get older, especially after age 60, the prostate may become a source of problems. Some of these problems are prostate cancer, an enlarged prostate (benign prostatic hyperplasia, or BPH), and prostatitis (inflammation of the prostate). The present Emperor had prostate cancer. Early diagnosis is especially important in prostate cancer. The prostate-specific antigen (PSA) is a protein made only by prostate cells. High PSA levels in the blood may be a sign of

---

sexually transmitted disease (STD, 性感染症)

infertility（不妊症）

development（発育）
deliver（分娩する）
sterility（不妊症）
ovulate（排卵する）

IVF (in vitro fertilization, 体外受精)
GIFT (gamete intra fallopian transfer, 卵管内配偶子移植法)

prostate（前立腺）

benign prostatic hyperplasia (BPH, 前立腺肥大)
prostatitis（前立腺炎）
the present Emperor（今上天皇）

prostate-specific antigen (PSA, 前立腺特異抗原)

Chapter 10

prostate cancer. Men over 50 years old should have a PSA test and digital rectal examination (DRE) once a year.

digital rectal examination (DRE, 指触診古腸検査)

Breast and uterine cancers are probably the most common cancer among women. In Japan, the mortality rate of uterine cancer has declined gradually, but death from breast cancer has increased from 9.4% in 1990 to 14.9% in 2002. One of the strongest risk factors for breast cancer may be old age. Doctors recently found that some cancers are related to mutations (changes in the genes) in either the gene BRCA1 or BRCA2. After 50 years old, women should have a yearly mammogram, an X-ray of the breast.

breast cancer(乳がん)
uterine cancer(子宮がん)
mortality(死亡率)

mutations(突然変異)
gene(遺伝子)

mammogram(乳房X線写真)

Questions 10(b)

Choose the best word from the list and fill in the blank.

1. If a man's sperm can not fertilize the woman's egg, he is _____.
2. If a woman can not ovulate, we say she is _____.
3. As men get older, especially after age 60, the _____ may become a source of problems.
4. _____ is a protein made only by the prostate cells.
5. The mortality rate of _____ cancer has declined gradually.
6. Old age may be one of the strongest _____ factors for breast cancer.
7. Doctors lately found that some breast cancers are related to _____ in some gene.

prostate	infertile	mutations	breast	sterile
risk	PSA	uterine		

101

Chapter 10

Vocabulary

benign prostatic hypertrophy (BPH) (prostatomegaly)	前立腺肥大
prostate cancer	前立腺がん
testicular tumor	精巣腫瘍
gynecomastia	女性化乳房
cervical carcinoma (cervical cancer)	子宮頸がん
endometrial carcinoma (corpus cancer)	子宮体がん
endometrial hyperplasia	子宮内膜増殖症（過形成）
myoma uteri (uterine leiomyoma)	子宮筋腫（子宮平滑筋腫）
ovarian tumor	卵巣腫瘍
choriocarcinoma	絨毛がん
fibroadenoma	線維腺腫
mastopathy	乳腺症
mastitis	乳腺炎，乳房炎
breast cancer	乳がん
sexually transmitted disease (STD)	性感染症
gonorrhea	淋病
syphilis	梅毒
lymphogranuloma venereum	鼠径リンパ肉芽腫症
trichomonas vaginitis	トリコモナス腟炎
climacteric disturbance	更年期障害
infertility	不妊症
artificial fertilization	人工受精
in vitro fertilization (IVF)	体外受精
amniocentesis	羊水穿刺

Chapter 10

接尾辞

接尾辞	意味	例
-ia	～症（病気の状態）	gynecomastia
-itis	～炎（炎症）	mastitis
-megaly	肥大，巨大	prostatomegaly
-oma	腫瘍，新生物	carcinoma, fibroadenoma, leiomyoma lymphogranuloma
-pathy	病気	mastopathy
-plasia	形成	hyperplasia
-trophy	栄養	hypertrophy

生殖器系の語根

語根の連結形	意味
orch/o, orchi/o, orchid/o	精巣（testis）
scrot/o	陰嚢（scrotum）
phall/o	陰茎（penis）
prostat/o	前立腺（prostate）
sperm/o, spermat/o, sperm/i	精子（sperm）
oo/o	卵（ovum）
oophor/o, ovari/o	卵巣（ovary）
salping/o	卵管（salpinx）
uter/o, hyster/o, metr/a, metr/o	子宮（uterus）
men/o	月経（menstruation）
cervic/o	子宮頸部（cervix）
colp/o, vagin/a	腟（vagina）
gyne, gynec/o	女性（woman）
placent/o	胎盤（placenta）
chori/o	絨毛膜（membrane）
amni/o	羊膜（amnion）
fet/o	胎児（fetus）
mamm/o, mast/o	乳房（breast）
lact/o, lact/i, galact/o	乳汁（lactis）

Chapter 10

練習問題 10

1. -itis（炎症）とつないで次の用語をつくりなさい。
   1. 精巣炎 _____
   2. 前立腺炎 _____
   3. 子宮頸管炎 _____
   4. 子宮内膜炎 _____
   5. 乳腺炎（乳房炎）_____
   6. 腟炎 _____

2. -ectomy（切除術）とつないで次の用語をつくりなさい。
   1. 精巣摘除（術）_____
   2. 陰嚢切除（術）_____
   3. 精管切除（術）_____
   4. 前立腺切除（術）_____
   5. 卵巣摘出（術）_____
   6. 子宮摘出（術）_____

3. -otomy（切開術）を含む次の用語の意味をいいなさい。
   1. orchiotomy(orchidotomy) _____
   2. prostatocystotomy _____

4. mammo-，masto-（乳房）を含む次の用語の意味をいいなさい。
   1. mammography _____
   2. mammoplasty _____
   3. mastography _____
   4. mastectomy _____

5. 子宮（hystero-）を含む次の用語をつくりなさい。
   1. 子宮鏡 _____
   2. 子宮鏡検査 _____
   3. 子宮造影（法）_____
   4. 子宮造影図 _____

6. spermato-（精子）または oo-（卵）を含む次の用語の意味をいいなさい。
   1. spermatocyte _____
   2. spermatogenesis _____
   3. oocyte _____
   4. oogenesis _____

7. -cele（〜のヘルニア）を含む次の用語の意味をいいなさい。
   1. orchiocele _____
   2. hysterocele _____
   3. ovariocelle _____
   4. salpingocele _____
   5. salpingo-oophorocele _____
   6. vaginocele _____

8. 次の用語の意味をいいなさい。
   1. prostatomegaly _____
   2. aspermia _____
   3. oligospermia _____
   4. menopause _____
   5. gynecology _____
   6. obstetrics _____

Chapter 10

9．次の用語の意味をいいなさい。
生殖器系の略語

Ab, ab, abor	abortion	
AI	artificial insemination	
AID	artificial insemination with donor's semen	
BPH	benign prostate hypertrophy	
D&C	dilation and curettage	
DRE	digital rectal examination	
Gyn, GYN	gynecology	
in utero	within uterus	
IVF	in vitro fertilization in vivo fertilization	
LMP	last menstrual period	
Obs-Gyn	obstetrics and gynecology	
PSA	prostate-specific antigen	
PV	per vagina	
STD	sexually transmitted disease	
syph.	syphilis	
VE	vaginal examination	
WR	Wasserman reaction	

Chapter 11

Endocrine System
（内分泌系）

Overview

The body has two main systems for controlling all of its functions: the nervous system and the endocrine system. Unlike the quick effect of the nervous system, the endocrine system functions rather slowly and delicately. The endocrine system plays a crucial role in all important functions including growth, reproduction, metabolism and so on.

The hormones are chemical messengers which are secreted into the blood from ductless glands. Since the blood flows to every cell in the body, only cells which are sensitive to the hormone (have a receptor on their surface or inside the cell) will respond. These sensitive (hormone-specific) cells are also called target cells.

The most famous glands (and their hormones) are hypothalamus (TRH, CRH, GnRH, PRL-RH), pituitary (TSH, ACTH, FSH, LH, growth hormone, prolactin, vasopressin and oxytocin), thyroid (T_3, T_4 and calcitonin), parathyroid (parathormone), pancreas (insulin and glucagon), adrenal (epinephrine, norepinephrine, cortisol and aldosterone), testes (testosterone and estrogen), ovaries (estrogen, progesterone,

---

crucial（非常に重要な）
chemical messengers（化学伝達物質）
secrete（分泌する）
ductless glands（導管のない腺）
target cells（標的細胞）
hypothalamus（視床下部）
TRH（甲状腺刺激ホルモン放出ホルモン）
CRH（副腎皮質刺激ホルモン放出ホルモン）
GnRH 性腺刺激ホルモン放出ホルモン，ゴナドトロピン放出ホルモン）
PRL-RH（プロラクチン放出ホルモン）
pituitary gland（下垂体）
TSH（甲状腺刺激ホルモン）
ACTH（副腎皮質刺激ホルモン）
FSH（卵胞刺激ホルモン）
LH（黄体化ホルモン）
growth hormone（成長ホルモン）
prolactin（プロラクチン）
vasopressin（バソプレシン）
oxytocin（オキシトシン）

Chapter 11

testosterone).

The pituitary gland, the size of a pea, is considered the most important part of the endocrine system. It's often called the "master gland" because it makes hormones that control several other endocrine glands. The front part of the pituitary controls the thyroid, adrenals, and reproductive glands.

---

thyroid gland(甲状腺)
T_3(トリヨードサイロニン)
T_4(サイロキシン, チロキシン)
calcitonin(カルシトニン)
parathyroid glands(副甲状腺)
pancreas(膵臓)
insulin(インスリン)
glucagon(グルカゴン)
adrenal glands(副腎)
epinephrine(エピネフリン)
norepinephrine(ノルエピネフリン)
cortisol(コルチゾル)
aldosterone(アルドステロン)
testes(精巣)
testosterone(テストステロン)
estrogen(エストロゲン)
ovaries(卵巣)
progesterone(プロゲステロン)

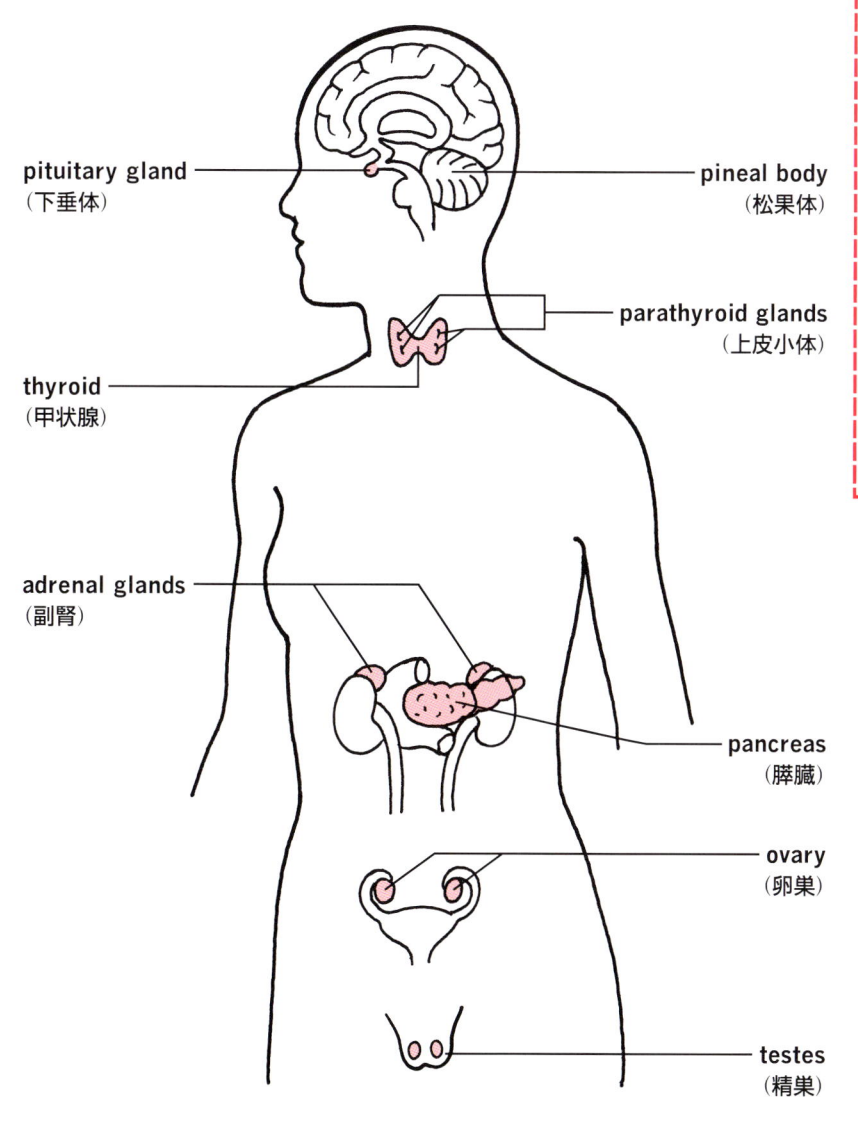

Fig 11-1 Endocrine system(内分泌系)

Chapter 11

Questions 11(a)

Choose the best word from the list and fill in the blank.

1. Unlike the quick effect of the _____ system, the _____ system works rather slowly and delicately.
2. The endocrine system plays a crucial role in growth, reproduction, _____ and so on.
3. The hormones are chemical _____ .
4. The hormones are secreted into the blood from _____ glands.
5. The cells which are sensitive to the hormone are called _____ cells.

metabolism	target	endocrine	nutrient	messengers
nervous	reproductive	ductless		

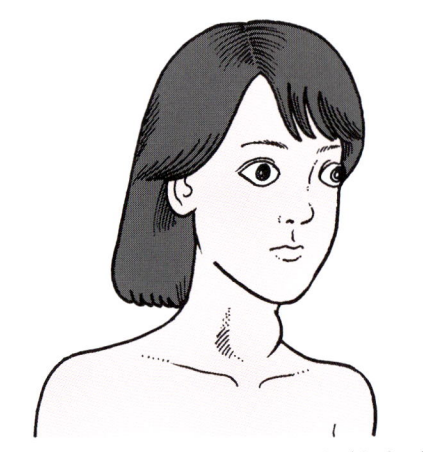

Fig 11-2 Basedow's disease(バセドウ病)

Chapter 11

Disorders of the Endocrine System
(内分泌系の疾患)

The most well known disease involving a hormone is diabetes mellitus (DM). It is a life-long disease marked by high levels of sugar (glucose) in the blood. Insulin is the hormone secreted by the pancreas that controls the level of sugar in the body. Diabetes is caused because the pancreas does not produce enough insulin or the body is not sensitive to insulin. It may be both of these problems together. There are two main types of diabetes: Type I diabetes (IDDM; insulin dependent diabetes mellitus) and Type II diabetes (NIDDM; non-insulin dependent diabetes mellitus). Type I diabetes occurs when we are children and Type II diabetes, the most common type, occurs in adults. Some of the symptoms of DM include increased thirst, increased urination and fatigue.

The thyroid is one of the most important glands of the endocrine system. Thyroid hormones regulate metabolism and body temperature, and are essential for normal growth and fertility. Graves' disease or Basedow's disease is the result of an overactive thyroid gland (hyperthyroidism). Too much thyroid hormone can lead to burnout. Women are more affected than men. People with Graves' disease seem nervous and over stimulated. Doctors aren't sure what triggers this problem, but they do know that the immune system is involved. In Graves' disease patients, they find special

---

diabetes mellitus (真性糖尿病)

diabetes (糖尿病)
Type I diabetes (インスリン依存型糖尿病)
Type II diabetes (インスリン非依存型糖尿病)

thirst (渇き)

urination (排尿)

fatigue (疲労)
thyroid (=thyroid gland 甲状腺)

fertility (生殖能力)
hyperthyroidism (甲状腺機能亢進症)
burnout (燃えつき)

trigger (引き金を引く)

Chapter 11

antibodies that stimulate the thyroid.

Cushing's syndrome is a disease caused by an excess (too much) cortisol or other similar steroid (glucocorticoid) hormones. Cortisol is a normal hormone produced in the outer part (cortex) of the adrenal glands which are located above each kidney. The function (job) of cortisol is to help the body respond to stress and stress-induced physiological change. Cortisol also helps to regulate nutrients in the body and control the body's response to inflammation. Cortisol stimulates the liver to raise the blood sugar, and it helps control the amount of water in the body. Aldosterone is another hormone secreted from the adrenal cortex. It regulates salt and water levels which affect (influence) blood volume and blood pressure. Some symptoms of Cushing's syndrome include hypertension, obesity, muscle wasting, thin skin, and diabetes.

antibodies（抗体）
stimulate（刺激する）
cortex（皮質）
induce（ひき起こす）
inflammation（炎症）
secrete（分泌する）
obesity（肥満）
wasting（衰弱）

Questions 11(b)

Choose the best word from the list and fill in the blank.

1. Insulin is secreted by the _____.
2. _____ is caused because the pancreas does not produce enough insulin or the body is not sensitive to insulin.
3. _____ is the result of an overactive thyroid gland.
4. _____ is a disease caused by an excess of cortisol.
5. Cortisol and aldosterone are produced in the outer part (cortex) of the _____.

diabetes mellitus	adrenal glands	cortex	Cushing's syndrome
Basedow's disease	pancreas	thyroid	

Chapter 11

Vocabulary

giantism	巨人症
acromegaly	末端肥大症
dwarfism	小人症
Simmonds' disease	シモンズ病
diabetes insipidus	尿崩症
goiter	甲状腺腫
hyperthyroidism	甲状腺機能亢進症
Basedow's disease (Graves' disease)	バセドウ病(グレーブス病)
hypothyroidism	甲状腺機能低下症
cretinism	クレチン病
myx(o)edema	粘液水腫
Hashimoto thyroiditis (chronic thyroiditis)	橋本病(慢性甲状腺炎)
autoimmune thyroiditis	自己免疫性甲状腺炎
hyperparathyroidism	副甲状腺機能亢進症
hypoparathyroidism	副甲状腺機能低下症
tetany (carpopedal spasm)	テタニー(四肢の強直性痙攣)
Cushing's syndrome	クッシング症候群
primary aldosteronism (Conn syndrome)	原発性アルドステロン症 (コン症候群)
chronic adrenal cortex insufficiency (Addison's disease)	慢性副腎皮質機能低下症 (アジソン病)
pheochromocytoma	褐色細胞腫
neuroblastoma	神経芽細胞腫
multiple endocrine neoplasia (MEN)	多発性内分泌腺腫症
diabetes mellitus (DM)	糖尿病
type 1 insulin-dependent diabetes mellitus (IDDM)	1型インスリン依存性糖尿病
type 2 non-insulin-dependent diabetes mellitus (NIDDM)	2型非インスリン依存性糖尿病

Chapter 11

ketoacidosis	ケトアシドーシス
coma	昏睡
diabetic macroangiopathy	糖尿病性大血管症
diabetic microangiopathy	糖尿病性細血管症
hypoglycemia	低血糖症

接頭辞・接尾辞

接頭・接尾	意味	例
acro-	先端	acromegaly
hyper-	過剰，正常範囲を超えている	hyperthyroidism
hypo-	欠乏，正常以下	hypothyroidism hypoglycemia
para-	近傍の	hyperparathyroidism
-itis	～炎（炎症）	thyroiditis
-megaly	肥大，巨大	acromegaly
-oma	腫瘍，新生物	pheochromocytoma neuroblastoma
-osis	～症（病気の過程, 状況, 状態）	ketoacidosis
-pathy	～症，～療法	macroangiopathy microangiopathy
-plasia	形成	neoplasia

Chapter 11

内分泌系の語根

語根の連結形	意味
adren/o, adrenal/o	副腎(adrenal glands)
adrenocortic/o	副腎皮質(adrenal cortex)
andr/o	男性(men, male)
calc/o	カルシウム(calcium)
cortic/o	皮質(cortex)
gluc/o, glyc/o	ブドウ糖(glucose), 糖(sugar)
gonad/o	性腺(gonad)
kal/i	カリウム(potassium)
lact/o	乳汁(milk)
myx/o	粘液(mucus)
natr/o	ナトリウム(sodium)
pancreat/o	膵臓(pancreas)
somat/o	体(body)
thyr/o, thyroid/o	甲状腺(thyroid gland)
pituitar-	下垂体(pituitary gland)

Chapter 11

練習問題11

1. アルドステロン産生の障害により生じる次の疾患を日本語にしなさい。
   1. hypernatremia _____
   2. hypokalemia _____
   3. natriuresis _____

2. insulin を含む次の用語の意味を言いなさい。
   1. insulinitis _____
   2. insulinoma _____
   3. insulinogenesis _____
   4. hyperinsulinism _____

3. 糖尿病に関連する次の症状・疾患を日本語にしなさい。
   1. hyperglycemia _____
   2. glycosuria _____
   3. polydipsia _____
   4. polyuria _____
   5. ketoacidosis _____
   6. coma _____
   7. diabetic macroangiopathy _____
   8. diabetic microangiopathy _____

4. 次のホルモンを産生する内分泌腺を下記のリストから選んで記入しなさい。
   1. adrenaline (epinephrine) _____
   2. cortisol _____
   3. estrogen _____
   4. insulin _____
   5. testosterone _____
   6. thyroxin _____

   | pancreatic islets | thyroid gland | testes | pituitary gland |
   | adrenal medulla | ovaries | adrenal cortex |

Chapter 11

5．日本語の意味を調べなさい。
内分泌系の略語

ACTH	adrenocorticotropic hormone	
ADH	antidiuretic hormone	
CRH	corticotropin releasing hormone	
FBS	fasting blood sugar	
FSH	follicle-stimulating hormone	
GH	growth hormone	
GnRH	gonadotropin releasing hormone	
GTT	glucose tolerance test	
hCG	human chorionic gonadotropin	
IDDM	insulin-dependent diabetes mellitus	
LH	luteinizing hormone	
LHRH	luteinizing hormone releasing hormone	
MEN	multiple endocrine neoplasia	
NIDDM	non-insulin-dependent diabetes mellitus	
PRL	prolactin level	
PTH	parathyroid hormone	
TSH	thyroid-stimulating hormone	
T_3	triiodothyronine	
T_4	thyroxine	

Part II Examinations and Treatments
（検査と処置）

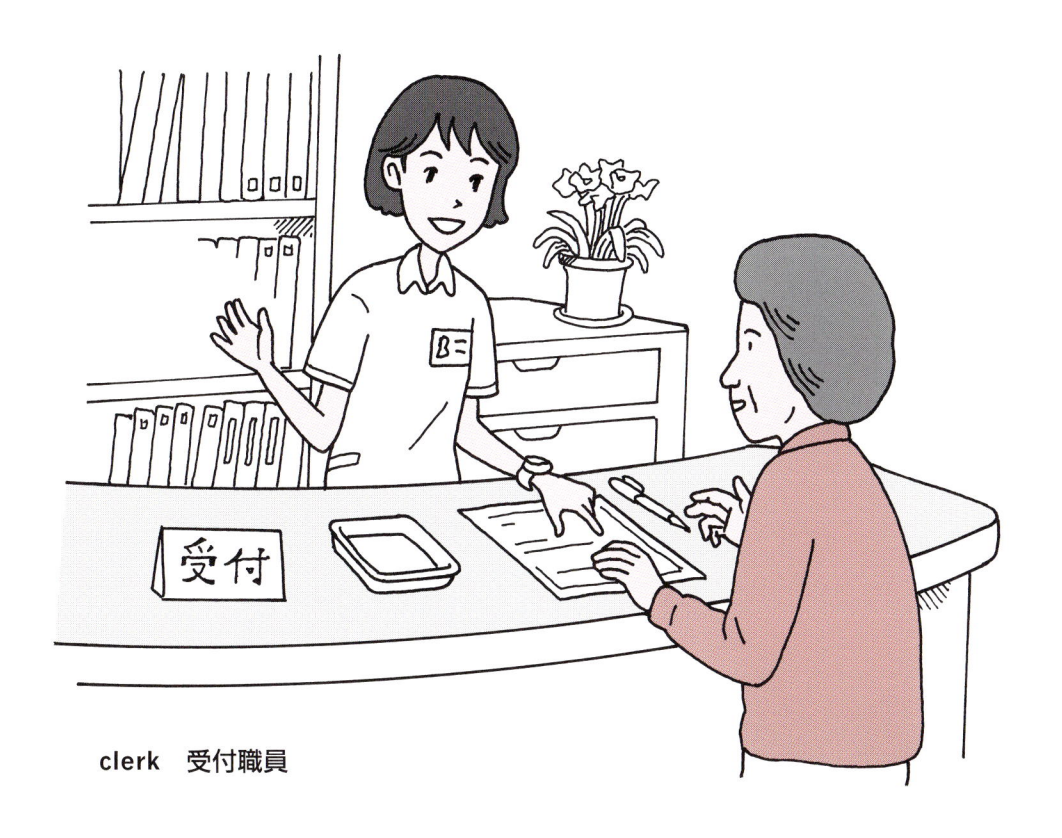

clerk　受付職員

Chapter 12

Examinations―検査

1. Blood Tests―血液検査
2. Vital Signs―バイタルサイン
3. Electrocardiography (ECG)―心電図検査
4. Endoscopy―内視鏡検査
5. Ultrasonography―超音波検査
6. X-ray Examination―X 線検査
7. Magnetic Resonance Imaging (MRI)―磁気共鳴画像法
8. Biopsy (BX)―生検

Chapter 12-1

Blood Tests
（血液検査）

The blood test (also called lab test) measures many different things in the blood. Doctors know the average values of these things in the blood of healthy people. We call this the normal level. For example, we know that there are about 7,000 white blood cells in each (per) cubic millimeter (mm^3) of blood. If someone's blood test shows that their level is higher than normal, we can guess they have an infection.

cubic millimeter（立方ミリメーター, mm^3）

infection（感染）

Blood is usually taken from the arm. A needle is put into (inserted) a vein.

insert（挿入する）

vein（静脈）

In the Blood Lab

Health Care Professional (HCP):
　　Please put your arm here and make a fist.

fist（握りこぶし）

Patient (P): OK.

HCP: You may feel just a little pain.
　　Please open your hand. You can relax.

HCP: Hold this (cotton) on the spot for five minutes.
　　Then put this (bandage) on.

Chapter 12-1

Blood Tests 検査項目	略号	基準値
Red blood cell count 赤血球数	RBC	$400〜550 \times 10^4/\mu L$ （男） $380〜500 \times 10^4/\mu L$ （女）
Hemoglobin 血色素量(ヘモグロビン量)	Hb	$14〜18$ g/dL （男） $12〜16$ g/dL （女）
Hematocrit ヘマトクリット	Ht	$36〜50\%$ （男） $30〜45\%$ （女）
Mean corpuscular volume 平均赤血球容積	MCV	$86〜98$(fL)
Mean corpuscular hemoglobin 平均赤血球血色素量	MCH	$27〜35$(pg)
Mean corpuscular hemoglobin concentration 平均赤血球色素濃度	MCHC	$31〜35(\%)$
White blood cell count 白血球数	WBC	$3,500〜9,000/\mu L$
Platelet count 血小板数	PL	$13〜40 \times 10^4/\mu L$
Bleeding time 出血時間		$2〜5$ min
Prothrombin time プロトロンビン時間	PT	$11〜15$ sec
Activated partial thromboplastin time 活性化部分トロンボプラスチン時間	APTT	$25〜45$ sec
Fibrinogen (mg/dL) フィブリノーゲン		$200〜400$ mg/dL
Fibrinogen degradation products フィブリノーゲン分解産物	FDP	$2.0〜8.0\,\mu g/mL$

Chapter 12-2

Vital Signs
（バイタルサイン）

The three most important vital signs are temperature, pulse and blood pressure. In CCU/ICU, vital signs are monitored continuously by machines including electrocardiograph, pulse oximeter, sphygmomanometer, etc.

electrocardiograph
（心電計）

pulse oximeter
（パルスオキシメーター）

sphygmomanometer
（血圧計）

Conversation

Health Care Professional (HCP):
　　I would like to check your vital signs now. What is your blood pressure usually?

Patient (P): It's usually about 125 over 70. How is it now?

HCP: Now it is 130 over 75. You might be a little nervous today. It is in the normal level so that there is no problem. Your temperature is also normal. But your pulse seems a little high. Do you smoke?

P:　Yes, I do. What is my pulse now?

HCP: It's 84. The normal range is anywhere from 55 to 75 when we are resting. We will check to see if there are any problems. Don't worry

Notes: CCU (critical care unit, 重症患者集中治療室；coronary care unit＝冠疾患集中治療室の意もある)
　　　ICU (intensive care unit, 集中治療室)

Chapter 12-2

Vocabulary

vital signs	バイタルサイン，生命兆候
pulse rate	脈拍数
respiratory rate	呼吸数
blood pressure (BP)	血圧
systolic blood pressure (SBP)	収縮期血圧
diastolic blood pressure (DBP)	拡張期血圧
body temperature	体温
consciousness	意識レベル
oxygen saturation	酸素飽和度
thermometer	体温計
by mouth, orally	口腔による
by armpit, axillary	腋窩による
by rectum, rectally	直腸による
emergency room (ER)	救急救命室
lifesaver	救命士
ambulance	救急車

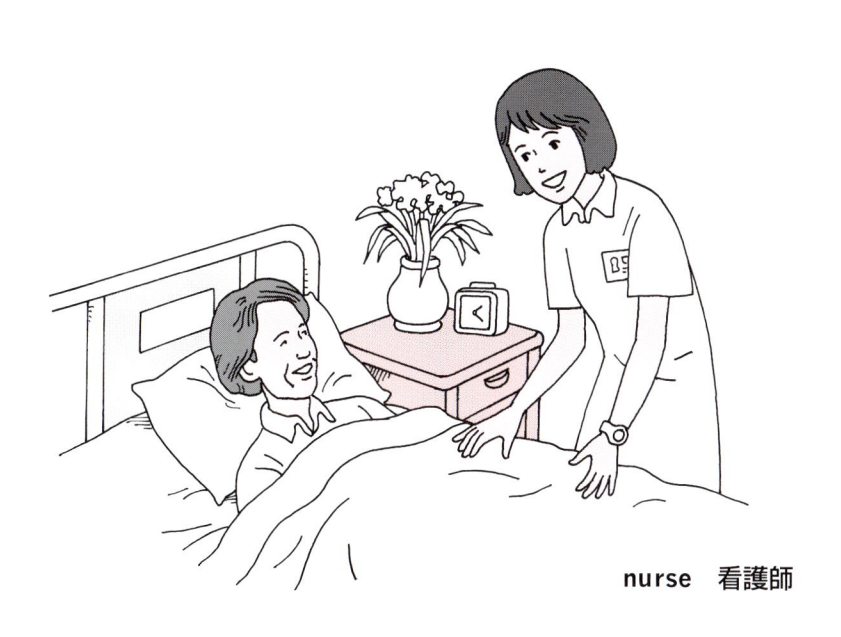

nurse 看護師

Chapter 12-3

Electrocardiography (ECG)
(心電図検査)

ECG comes from the three Greek words, electricity *(electro)*, heart *(cardio)* and write *(graphy)*. We can measure the activities of the heart electrically.

An electrocardiogram gives us a graphical picture of the different parts (phases) of the heartbeat. An ECG record when the patient is resting may show that the blood supply of the heart appears to be normally maintained. Sometimes the patient does some exercise like walking on a treadmill or riding a stationary bicycle. This is called a stress test. As the exercise increases, the doctor looks for changes in the ECG which show (indicate) that the heart is not getting enough oxygen.

heartbeat (心臓の鼓動, 拍動)
resting (休息している)
exercise (運動)
treadmill (トレッドミル)
stationary (動かない, 静止した)

In the Lab

Health Care Professional (HCP):
　　We are going to attach some wires to your chest and ankles. Please remove your clothes in those areas. Lie down here and make yourself comfortable.

Patient (P): This is my first time and I am a little nervous.

HCP: There is no pain. It is a very easy exam and only takes a few minutes. We finished the exam. You may put on your clothes and sit in the waiting room.

wire (針金, ワイヤー)
chest (胸)
ankle (足首)

Chapter 12-3

Vocabulary

electrocardiograph (ECG, EKG)	心電計
electrocardiogram (ECG, EKG)	心電図
resting ECG	安静時心電図
stress ECG	負荷心電図
treadmill testing	トレッドミル負荷試験法
Holter ECG	ホルター心電図
artificial pacemaker ECG	人工ペースメーカー ECG
cardiac cycle	心臓周期
heart rate	心拍数
systole	収縮期
diastole	拡張期
heart sound	心音
cardiac output	心拍出量
stroke volume	1回拍出量

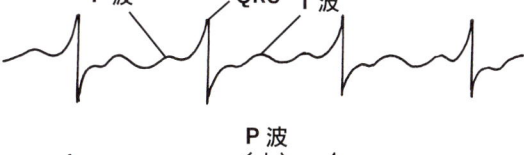

normal ECG
(正常心電図)

complete AV block
(完全房室ブロック)

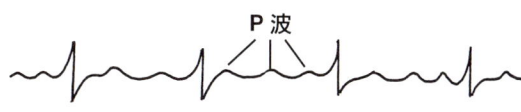

atrial flutter
(心房粗動)

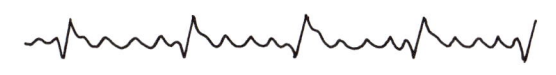

atrial fibrillation
(心房細動)

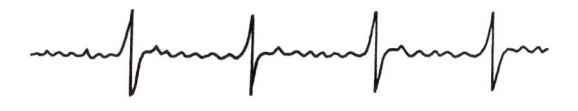

ventricular tachycardia
(心室頻脈)

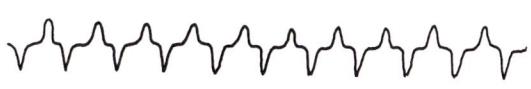

ventricular fibrillation
(心室細動)

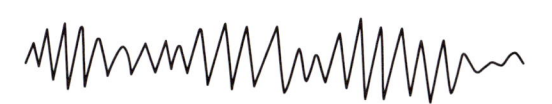

Fig 12-1 Electrocardiogram(心電図)

Chapter 12-4

Endoscopy
（内視鏡検査）

The endoscope is a flexible tube which we can put down the mouth or up the anus to look at the inside of the digestive tract. There is a camera and scalpel. With the scalpel the doctor can cut out some small part of the digestive tract tissues that may have a problem, like a polyp.

flexible（曲げやすい）
anus（肛門）
digestive tract（消化管）
scalpel（外科用メス）
tissue（組織）
polyp（ポリープ）

GI Exam

GI exam（胃腸検査）

Health Care Professional (HCP):
We are going to put this tube down your throat to look at your stomach.

throat（のど）

Patient (P): Will it hurt?

HCP: It might feel a little uncomfortable at first, so we will let you gargle this medicine. So you won't gag.

uncomfortable（不快な）
gargle（うがいする）
medicine（薬）
gag（ゲーゲーする）

P: I'm nervous.

HCP: That is normal, but everything will be OK. It will be over in about 30 minutes. You can watch the TV monitor and I will explain what we are looking at.

Notes: GI exam (gastrointestinal examination, 胃腸検査)

Chapter 12-4

Vocabulary

endoscope	内視鏡
fiberscope	ファイバースコープ
gastroscope	胃鏡
gastroenteroscope	胃腸鏡
sigmoidoscope	S状結腸鏡
colonoscope	結腸鏡
proctoscope	直腸鏡
laparoscope	腹腔鏡
hysteroscope	子宮鏡
colposcope	腟鏡

接尾語

接尾辞	意味	例
-scope	視診するための機械（鏡）	gastroscope
-scopy	視覚的検査法	gastroscopy

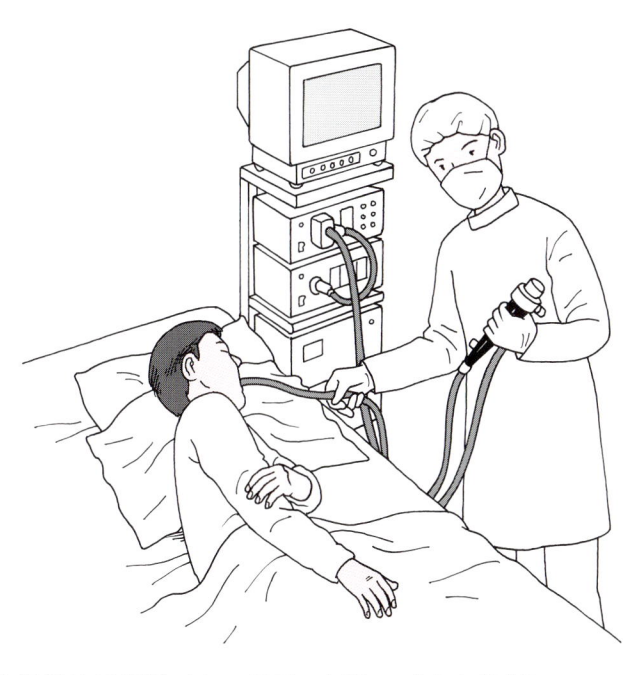

内視鏡は早期胃がんの発見・切除に威力を発揮している。

Chapter 12-5

Ultrasonography
(超音波検査)

Ultrasonography (echography) uses sound waves, so it is completely safe. The test is quick and painless for the patient. One of the most common uses is to look at a baby inside a mother's womb (uterus).

OB/GYN Exam of Pregnant Woman

Health Care Professional (HCP):
　　We are going to look at the baby using ECHO.

Patient (P): I've heard about it.

HCP: It is very simple and safe. I am going to put this jelly on your belly first. Now you can see the baby on the TV. This is the head.

P: Can you tell if it is a boy or a girl?

HCP: It looks like a boy. Unless, it is a girl with her hand between her legs.

Notes: OB/GYN (obstetrics and gynecology, 産・婦人科)

sound wave（音波）	
womb（＝uterus 子宮）	
OB/GYN（産・婦人科）	
pregnant woman（妊婦）	
ECHO（超音波検査法）	
belly（腹部）	

Chapter 12-5

Vocabulary

ultrasonogram	超音波検査図
ultrasonograph	超音波検査装置
ultrasonography	超音波検査法
ultrasound scans	
echocardiogram	超音波心臓検査図
	(心臓エコー図)
echoencephalogram	超音波脳検査図
	(脳エコー図)
echoencephalograph	超音波脳検査装置

接尾辞

接尾辞	意味	例
-gram	記録，図	ultrasonogram, electrocardiogram
-graph	(記録する)装置	ultrasonograph, electrocardiograph
-graphy	記録法	ultrasonography, electrocardiography

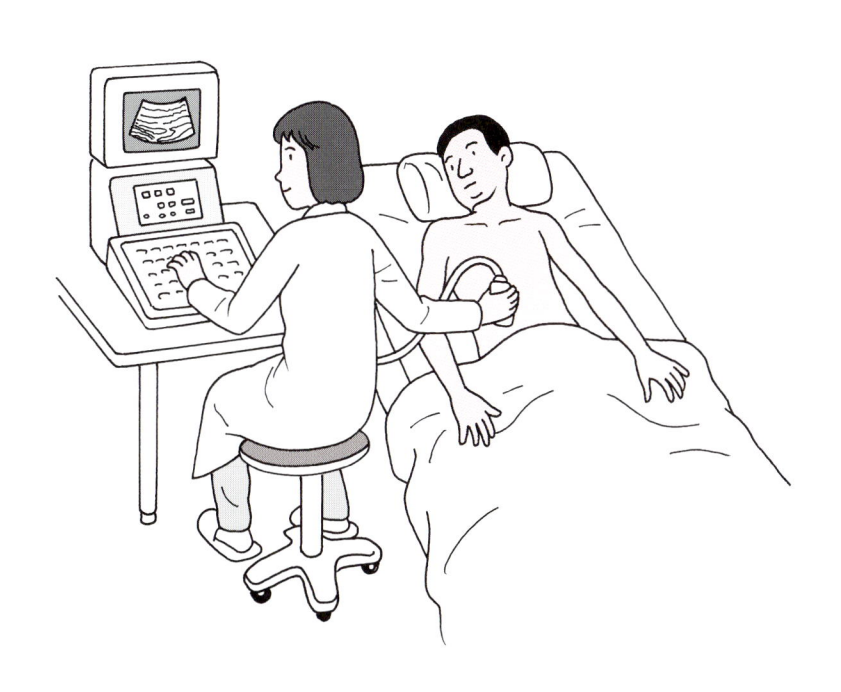

Chapter 12-6

X-ray Examination
（X 線検査）

X-ray photographs, called radiographs, are used very often in clinical medicine as diagnostic tools.　X-rays can go through our body in different amounts and let us know problems inside our body.　X-ray can be dangerous if we get too much. Computed tomography (CT) scanning uses X-rays.　It takes many different layers of pictures (slices) and a computer saves all the slices and puts together a three dimensional (3-D) picture.

diagnostic tool（診断法）

layer（層）
slice（薄切り）
three-dimensional
（3 次元の）

Health Care Professional (HCP): Please take off your upper clothes and put on this robe.　I will call you soon.

Patient (P): Do I wait here?

HCP: Yes.　Please sit over there.

robe（ローブ）

In the X-ray Room

HCP: Please put your chest against the machine.

P:　　Like this?

HCP: That's right.　And put your chin on this part.

P:　　Right here?

HCP: Yes.　That's fine.　Now take a deep breath and hold it.

chest（胸）

chin（あご）

Chapter 12-6

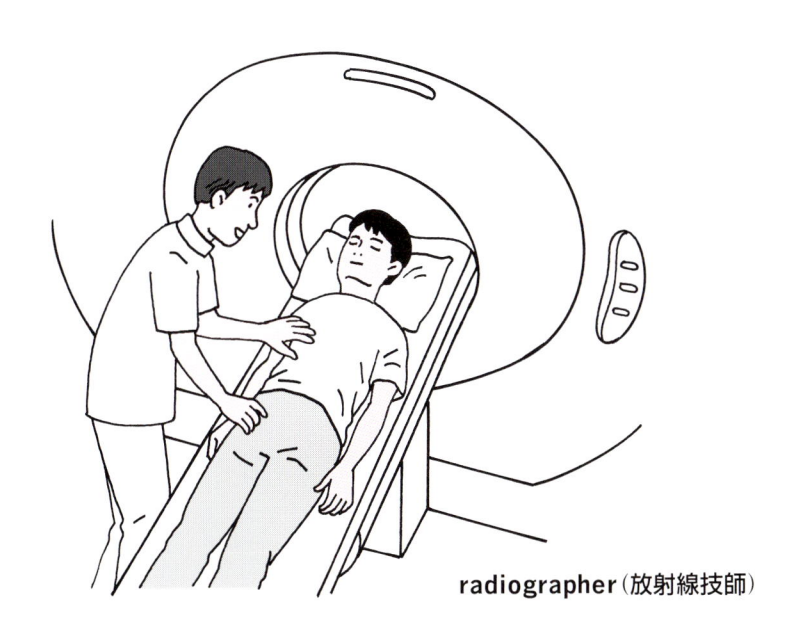

HCP: You can relax now.　We finished our exam.　You can go and change.

Vocabulary

radiologist	放射線科医
radiogram	X線写真
radiography	X線撮影(法)
radiographer	X線撮影技師
radiotherapy	放射線治療(法)
radiotherapist	放射線治療医
cineradiography	シネラジオグラフィー
cineangiography	血管映画撮影(法)
cineangiocardiography	血管心臓映画撮影(法)
barium enema	注腸バリウム
tomography	断層X線撮影(法)
computed tomography (CT)	コンピュータ断層撮影(法)
CT scanning, CAT scanning	CTスキャン
positron emission tomography (PET)	陽電子放射断層撮影(法)
videofluorography (VF)	嚥下造影検査(法)

radiographer(放射線技師)

Chapter 12-7

Magnetic Resonance Imaging (MRI)
(磁気共鳴画像法)

Magnetic resonance imaging is a safe diagnostic technique. It uses a strong magnetic field and radio waves rather than harmful dyes or x-rays.　MRI images create several "slices of an organ or part of the body".　The computer can combine these slices into 3-D images.　MRI is particularly important in detecting tumors and in checking for abnormalities in the body's soft tissues, such as the brain, spinal cord, heart and eye.

magnetic field（磁場）	
radio waves（電磁波）	
dye（造影剤）	
3-D（三次元の；D は dimensional の略）	
detect（検出する）	
tumor（腫瘍）	
abnormalities（異常）	

Health Care Professional (HCP): Do you have a pacemaker or any metal in your body, like an artificial joint?

Patient (P): No, I don't.

HCP: Good.

HCP: If you have to use the toilet, please go now.

P:　No.　I am OK.

HCP: Then go into this room and take off your clothes except underwear and socks.　Put on this robe with the open part in the back.　Then come out and sit here.

artificial joint（人工関節）

Chapter 12-7

In MRI Room

HCP: Please lie down on your back with your head here. The MRI is quite noisy. So please use these earplugs.

P: Is this OK?

HCP: Just fine. It will take about 30 minutes and it is quite small inside the machine. If you feel nervous or uncomfortable, please push this button and we will stop.

P: This red button at the end of the cord?

HCP: That's right.

Afterword

HCP: We finished our exam. Please go in the room and change.

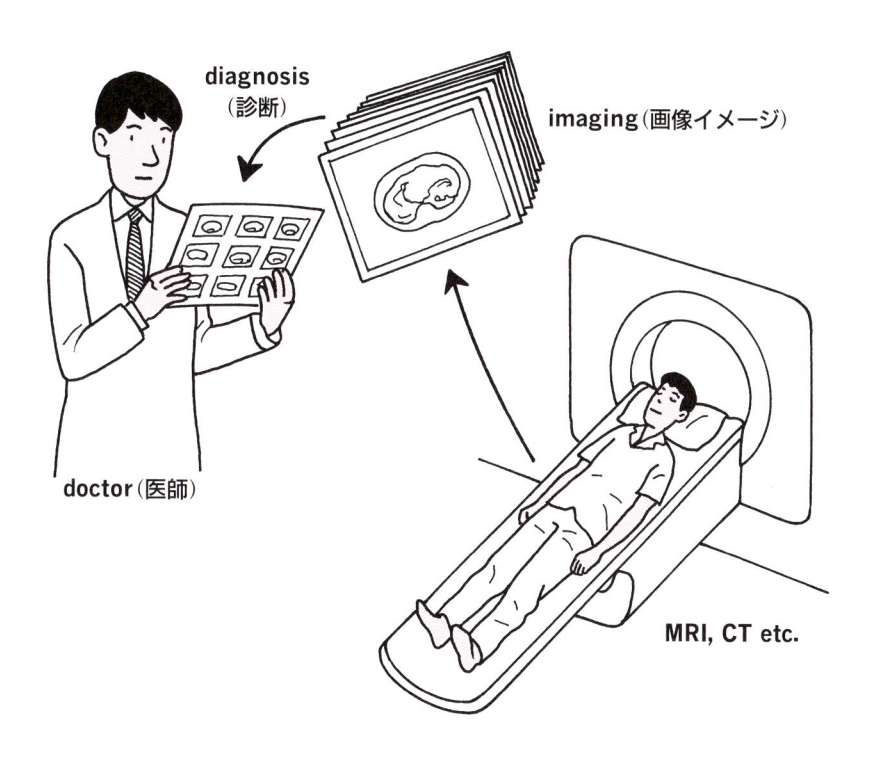

earplug（耳栓）

uncomfortable（不快な）

diagnosis（診断）
imaging（画像イメージ）
doctor（医師）
MRI, CT etc.

Chapter 12-8

Biopsy (BX)
(生検)

The word biopsy comes from *bio* which means life and *ops* meaning eye. A biopsy is performed when we take some tissues from a living body and look at it very closely to see what is making the problem. We usually use a microscope. There are two common ways to get the tissue. We can open the body with surgery. Or, we can use a long thin needle. The needle is hollow so that some tissues (cells) will be captured inside. This is called a needle or plug biopsy.

perform（行う）

microscope（顕微鏡）
tissue（組織）
surgery（手術）
thin needle（細い針）
hollow（中空の）

Needle Biopsy of Liver

Health Care Professional (HCP): I am going to put this needle into your liver and take out a small amount of cells.

Patient (P): Will it hurt much?

HCP: No, it won't. First, I will give you a few shots of painkiller. After a few minutes you will have no feeling in the area.

P: Will I have to stay in the hospital?

HCP: No. You will be able to leave in about two hours.

P: When should I come back?

HCP: We will get the information about your liver in two weeks. So you can come back then.

painkiller（鎮痛剤）

Chapter 12-8

Vocabulary

histological diagnosis	組織診，組織診検査
cytodiagnosis	細胞診，細胞診検査
biopsy	生検，生体組織検査法
autopsy (necropsy)	剖検，検死
tissue examination	組織検査
centesis	穿刺
smear	塗沫(標本)
pap smear	パップ塗沫標本
specimen	検体
histology	組織学
pathology	病理学
pathologist	病理学者
local anesthesia	局所麻酔

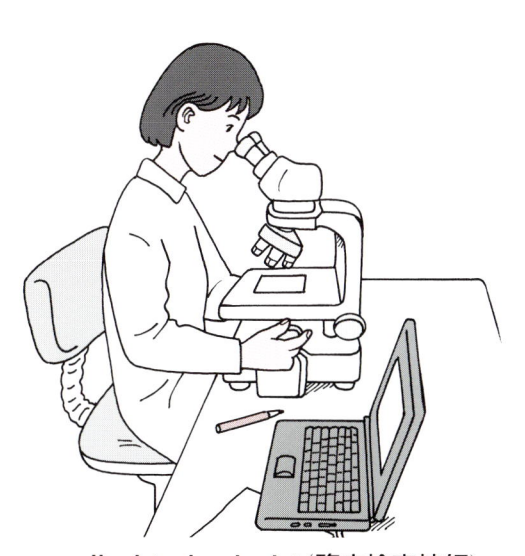

medical technologist(臨床検査技師)

Chapter 13
Treatments―処置

1. Intravenous (IV) Drip Infusion―点滴静注
2. Ventilator/Respirator―人工呼吸器
3. Hemodialysis―血液透析
4. Physical Therapy―理学療法
5. Occupational Therapy―作業療法
6. Dietetics/Nutrition―食事療法
7. Medication―薬物療法

Chapter 13-1

Intravenous (IV) Drip Infusion
(点滴静注)

The IV drip slowly puts medicine or fluid into the body. A needle is put (inserted) into a vein. The needle is connected to a tube that goes to a bag with the medicine or fluid (saline). The bag is usually hanging from a pole. There is no need to have any pump machine because gravity pulls the medicine downward. That is why the bag must always be higher than the needle. There is a little wheel connected to the tube. With the wheel we can control how fast the medicine goes into the tube.

insert (挿入する)
medicine (薬剤)
fluid (液体)
saline (生理食塩水)
pole (棒)
gravity (重力)
downward (下方へ)
wheel (車輪)

Health Care Professional (HCP):
　I am going to put a needle into your vein. This needle is connected to a tube that will drip medicine and fluid into your body. Which hand do you write with?

needle (針)

Patient (P): I am right-handed.

HCP: OK. We will use your left arm. This is tourniquet and I will tighten it. Please make a fist. The needle will hurt just a little.

tourniquet (止血帯)
fist (握りこぶし)

HCP: The tape will hold the needle in place so you can move your arm but don't over do it.

P: Do I have to stay in the bed?

Chapter 13-1

HCP: You can walk around but hold on to this pole with the drip bag.

HCP: I will check the drip often but if you notice that it is too slow or stops, please ring the bell and I will come.

P: OK. I understand.

Vocabulary

intravenous injection (i.v., IV)	静脈注射
intramuscular injection (i.m., IM)	筋肉注射
intracutaneous injection (i.c., IC)	皮内注射
(intradermal injection)	
subcutaneous injection (s.c., SC)	皮下注射
continuous intravenous drip infusion	点滴静注
(intravenous drip, i.v. drip)	
intravenous hyperalimentation	経静脈高カロリー輸液
(IVH)	（中心静脈栄養）
nasal tube feeding	経鼻経管栄養
catheter	カテーテル
catheterization	カテーテル挿入
cannula	カニューレ
cannulation, cannulization	カニューレ挿入
oral administration (peroral, p.o.)	経口投与
inhalation	吸入

Chapter 13-2

Ventilator/Respirator
(人工呼吸器)

Sometimes it is very difficult for a patient to breathe, so we use a machine to help him (her). This machine, called a ventilator (respirator), forces oxygen (O_2) into the lungs. The oxygen is sent in the same rhythm (synchronized) as the patient's breathing rate. Usually the patient is sedated (given medicine to sleep) so they are more comfortable.

breathe(呼吸する)
force(強要させる)
oxygen(酸素)
lung(肺)
rhythm(リズム)
synchronize(同時に発生する)
breathing rate(呼吸速度,呼吸数)
sedate(鎮静させる)
comfortable(快適な)

Health Care Professional (HCP):
  Because your father is unable to breathe well by himself, we are going to put him on the ventilator.

Family Member (FM): Will he be able to talk?

HCP: The ventilator is not so comfortable and patients try to fight it. So we will make him sleep and relax.

FM: How long will he have to stay on the machine?

HCP: We can't be sure. As soon as he can breathe well by himself, we will take him off the machine.

Chapter 13-2

Vocabulary

artificial breathing	人工呼吸
mouth-to-mouth technique	口対口人工呼吸法
exhaled air-ventilation method	呼気吹き込み法
breathing	呼吸
exhaling (expiration)	呼息(気)
inhaling (inspiration)	吸息(気)
heart-resuscitation technique	心蘇生法
heart massage	心臓マッサージ
cardiac compression technique	心臓圧迫法
home oxygen therapy (HOT)	在宅酸素療法
home mechanical ventilation (HMV)	在宅人工呼吸療法
trigger	トリガー(銃砲などの引き金)
ventilation	換気
assisted ventilation	補助換気
mechanical ventilation (MV)	機械換気
spontaneous ventilation	自発換気
weaning	ウィーニング(人工呼吸から離脱し自然呼吸に切り換えること;離乳法の意もある)
acidosis	アシドーシス
alkalosis	アルカローシス
acidemia	酸血症
alkalemia	アルカリ血症
baro-trauma	気圧障害
CO_2 narcosis	炭酸ガスナルコーシス
cyanosis	チアノーゼ
multiple organ failure (MOF)	多臓器不全
oxygen intoxication	酸素中毒
ventilation-associated pneumonia (VAP)	人工呼吸器関連肺炎
ventilator-induced lung injury (VILI) (ventilator-associated lung injury, VALI)	人工呼吸器関連肺障害

Chapter 13-2

peakflow meter		ピークフローメータ
pulse oxymeter		パルスオキシメータ
spirometer		スパイロメータ

呼吸管理に使われる記号・略号

A	alveolar	肺胞の
a	arterial	動脈(性)の
c	capillary	毛細血管の
v	venous	静脈(性)の
A-aDO$_2$	alveolar-arterial oxygen difference	肺胞気-動脈血酸素分圧較差
APRV	airway pressure release ventilation	気道内圧開放換気
BIPAP	biphasic positive airway pressure	二相性気道陽圧(バイパップ)
CPAP	continuous positive airway pressure	持続的気道陽圧(シーパップ)
CPPV	continuous positive pressure ventilation	持続陽圧換気
EIP	end-inspiratory pause	吸気終末休止期
FiO$_2$	fractional concentration of inspired oxygen	吸入気酸素濃度
FRC	functional residual capacity	機能的残気量
FVC	forced vital capacity	努力肺活量
HFV	high frequency ventilation	高頻度換気
IPPV	intermittent positive pressure ventilation	間欠的陽圧換気
IRV	inverse ratio ventilation	吸気/呼気時間逆転換気
NPPV	non-invasive positive pressure ventilation	非侵襲的陽圧換気
PAO$_2$	alveolar oxygen partial pressure	肺胞気酸素分圧
PaCO$_2$	arterial carbon dioxide partial pressure	動脈血二酸化炭素分圧

PaO$_2$	arterial oxygen partial pressure	動脈血酸素分圧
Paw	airway pressure	気道内圧
PEEP	positive end-expiratory pressure	終末呼気陽圧
PETCO$_2$	end-tidal carbon dioxide partial pressure	終末呼気二酸化炭素分圧
PSV	pressure support ventilation	圧支持換気
SaO$_2$	arterial oxygen saturation	動脈血酸素飽和度
SIMV	synchronized intermittent mandatory ventilation	同期式間欠的強制換気
SpO$_2$	oxygen saturation of peripheral arterial blood	末梢動脈血酸素飽和度
tcPO$_2$	transcutaneous oxygen partial pressure	経皮酸素分圧
tcPCO$_2$	transcutaneous carbon dioxide partial pressure	経皮二酸化炭素分圧
TV, VT	tidal volume	1回換気量
VC	vital capacity	肺活量
VD	dead space volume	死腔量

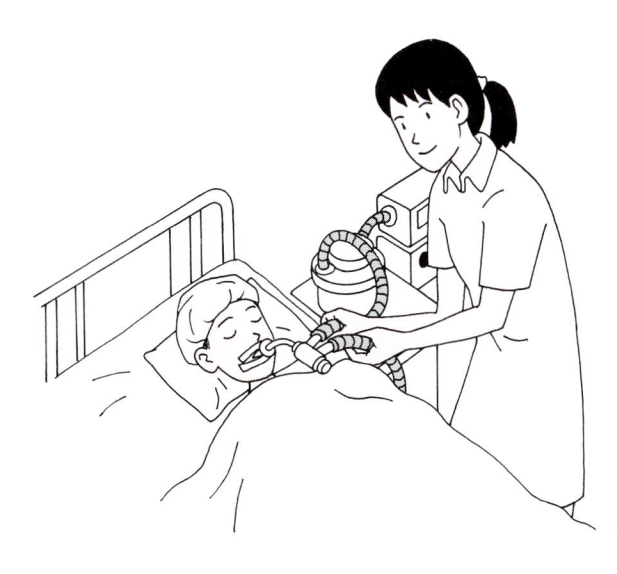

artificial breathing(人工呼吸)

Chapter 13-3

Hemodialysis
（血液透析）

Hemodialysis is used to treat patients with end-stage renal failure (ESRF).　In the session, blood is taken from the body, pumped into dialysis (kidney) machine, cleaned by an artificial kidney (dialyzer), and pumped back into the body.

end-stage renal failure（末期腎不全）

artificial kidney（人工腎臓）

Hemodialysis in Hospital

Health Care Professional (HCP):
    Please weigh yourself on the scales and then lie down on your back here.

HCP: I'm going to put a needle into your vein.　Just relax.　It won't hurt.

HCP: Please try not to move the arm connected to the machine.

HCP: I'm going to check your blood pressure and the machine every hour.　Let me know whenever you feel uncomfortable.

HCP: Your dialysis is over.　How are you feeling now?

Patient (P): I have a little cramp in my legs.

dialysis（透析）

cramp（痙攣）

Chapter 13-3

HCP: Well, we will give an injection of "Calcicol".

P: I feel better now. I think I am all right.

HCP: I'll take the needle out now and then I'll check your blood pressure and weight.

HCP: Please be careful what you eat and how much water you drink until your next dialysis.

P: I'm sure I will. Thank you.

Calcicol(カルチコール, カルシウム剤の商品名)

Vocabulary

hemodialysis (HD)	血液透析
hemofiltration (HF)	血液濾過
extracorporal ultrafiltration method (ECUM)	体外限外濾過法
hemodiafiltration (HDF)	血液透析濾過
continuous hemofiltration (CHF)	持続的血液濾過法
peritoneal dialysis (PD)	腹膜透析
intermittent peritoneal dialysis (IPD)	間欠的腹膜透析
continuous ambulatory peritoneal dialysis (CAPD)	持続式携帯型腹膜透析法
dialyzer	透析器
dialysis fluid, dialysate	透析液
dialysis membrane	透析膜
acid-base balance	酸・塩基平衡
air trap, bubble trap	気泡トラップ
air detector	気泡検出器
blood flow rate	(単位時間あたりの)血流速度
blood pump	血液ポンプ

Chapter 13-3

cardio thoracic ratio (CTR)	心胸比
convection	対流
diffusion	拡散
dry weight (DW)	ドライウエイト
electrolytes	電解質
erythropoietin (EPO)	エリスロポエチン
ethylene oxide gas (EOG)	エチレンオキサイドガス
extracorporal circulation	体外循環
excess water	過剰水分
fluid balance	体液平衡
fluid overload, overhydration	水分過剰
graft	移植組織
hemoabsorption	血液吸着
heparin pump	ヘパリンポンプ
negative pressure	陰圧
osmosis	浸透
plasma exchange	血漿交換
positive pressure	陽圧
protein catabolic rate (PCR)	タンパク異化率
recirculation	再循環
removal of water	除水
shunt	シャント，短絡
toxic waste	毒性老廃物
ultrafiltration	限外濾過
ultrafiltration rate (UFR)	限外濾過率
ultrafiltration pressure (TMP)	限外濾過圧（膜圧較差）
uremia	尿毒症
uremic toxins	尿毒症物質

Chapter 13-3

Possible Problems during hemodialysis(透析中に起こりやすい症状)

hypotension	低血圧
hypertension	高血圧
disequilibrium syndrome	不均衡症候群
cramps, spasm	痙攣
dizziness	めまい
unwell	気分のすぐれない
fever	発熱
fainting	気絶
chest pain	胸痛
headache	頭痛
vomiting	嘔吐
fatigue	疲労
irritability	怒りっぽいこと，過敏性
rigor, shivering attacks	硬直
restless legs syndrome	下肢静止不能症候群
burning feet syndrome	バーニングフィート(灼熱足)症候群
formication	蟻走感
anaphylaxis	アナフィラキシー

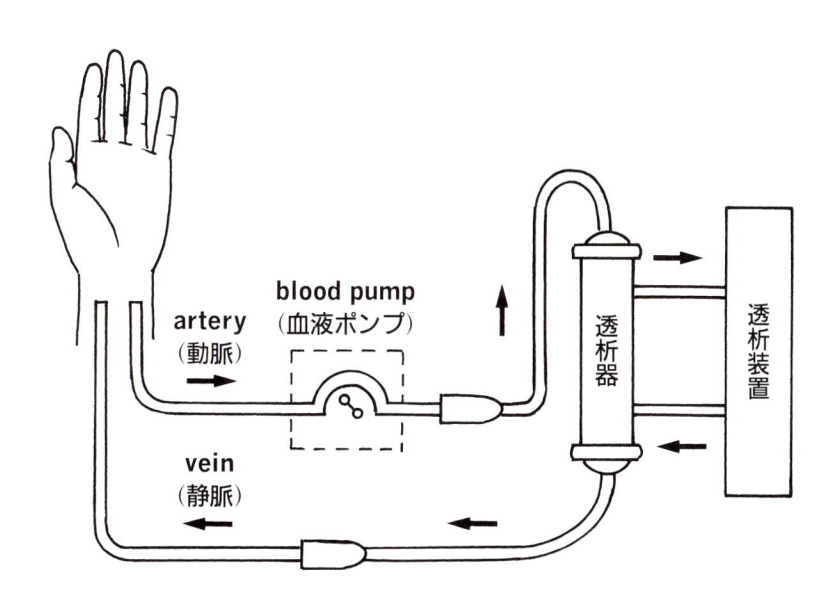

artery (動脈)
blood pump (血液ポンプ)
vein (静脈)
透析器
透析装置

Chapter 13-3

Possible complications(透析患者に起こりやすい合併症)

heart failure	心不全
hypertension	高血圧症
hyperkalemia	高カリウム血症
anemia	貧血
renal osteodystrophy (ROD)	腎性骨症，腎性骨異栄養症
infections	感染症
bleeding	出血(傾向)
amyloidosis	アミロイドーシス
carpal tunnel syndrome (CTS)	手根管症候群
pruritus (itching)	かゆみ，瘙痒

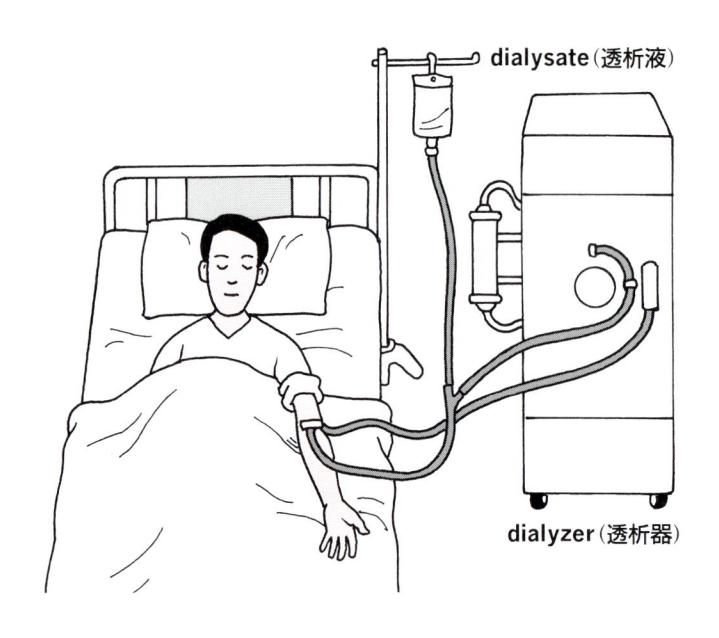

dialysate(透析液)

dialyzer(透析器)

Chapter 13-3

Possible Problems with the Shunt(シャントのトラブル)

shunt (arteriovenous shunt, A-V shunt)	シャント(動静脈シャント)
buzzing sensation	シャント音
thrill	スリル音
blocking by a blood clot	血液凝塊(血餅)による閉塞
bleeding	出血
infections	感染症
redness	発赤
swelling	腫脹

Other Useful Expressions

Check the buzzing thrill (sensation).	スリル(シャント音)を確かめてください。
Keep the shunt area clean.	シャント肢を清潔に保ってください。
Be careful to avoid infection to the shunt area.	シャント肢の感染に気をつけてください。

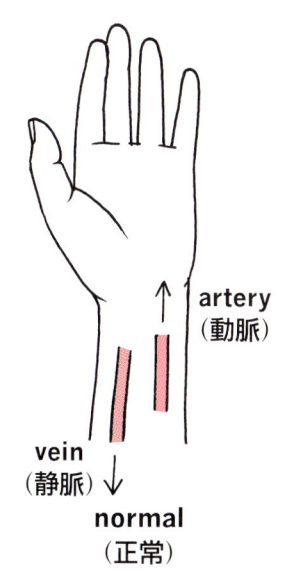

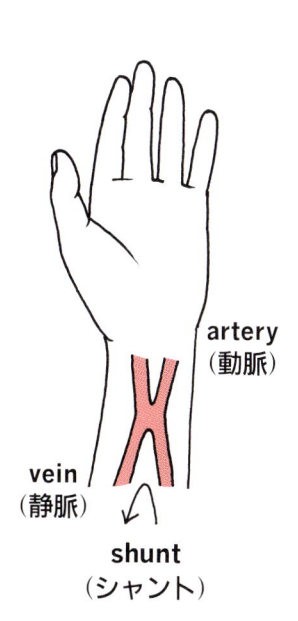

Chapter 13-4

Physical Therapy
(理学療法)

Therapists are people trained to rehabilitate patients through medical, physical, or occupational means. A physical therapist (PT) uses physical ways to help the patient. They use massage, heat, exercise and even electric current (diathermy) to help the senses and muscles work better. The most important thing for PT is to help the patient be able to take care of himself or herself.

physical(身体の, 肉体の)
therapist(療法士, セラピスト)
massage(マッサージ)
exercise(運動)
electric current(電流)
diathermy(ジアテルミー, 電気透熱)
sense(感覚)

Health care professional (HCP):
　　Today we are going to check on your leg strength. How does your leg feel?

Patient (P): I have trouble walking upstairs lately.

HCP: Sit here and push this pedal with your foot. We can measure how strong the muscle is.

P:　It does not seem too weak.

HCP: Let's change the weight. Please push.
　　OK. Let us begin some easy exercises for your leg.

Chapter 13-4

Vocabulary

physical therapist (PT)	理学療法士
physical therapy	物理療法，理学療法
actinotherapy	光線療法
diathermy	ジアテルミー
electrotherapy	電気療法
heat therapy	温熱療法
infrared therapy	赤外線療法
low frequency current therapy	低周波療法
traction treatment	牽引療法
ultrasound therapy	超音波療法
transcutaneous electrical nerve stimulation (TENS)	経皮的電気神経刺激
functional electrical stimulation (FES)	機能的電気刺激
therapeutic exercise	運動療法
active exercise	自動運動
passive exercise	他動運動
aerobic exercise	有酸素運動
anaerobic exercise	無酸素運動
assistance exercise	介助運動
breathing exercise	呼吸訓練
gait training	歩行訓練
muscle strengthening exercise	筋肉強化運動
postural exercise	姿勢(矯正)訓練
progressive resistance exercise	漸増抵抗運動
proprioceptive neuromuscular facilitation (PNF)	固有受容性神経筋肉促通法
range of motion exercise	(関節)可動域運動
massage	マッサージ
stretching	ストレッチング，伸張(法)
traction	牽引

Chapter 13-5

Occupational Therapy
(作業療法)

Occupational therapy uses the activities of everyday living to help people with physical or mental problems (disabilities). These activities usually use the hands, arms and legs to do things. Maybe the most important thing is using the mind to think and create. The patients often make craft items and play games.

mental(精神の)
disabilities
(単 disability 障害)
craft(手工芸)

Occupational Therapy Center (working with clay)

Health Care Professional (HCP):
　　Today we are going to make a cup out of clay.

clay(粘土)

Patient (P): I played with clay when I was a child in school.

HCP: Make a ball with the clay like this. Then push your thumb inside and press the sides.

thumb(親指)

P: Like this?

HCP: Yes. Try to squeeze the clay a little thinner and make it even. Now we can start to make it in the shape of a cup.

squeeze(しぼる)

P: The clay feels good in my hands but my fingers are a little stiff.

stiff(動きが悪い)

HCP: Well, this activity will help your hands and fingers to feel better. Next we will make the handle.

handle(柄, 取っ手)

Chapter 13-5

Vocabulary

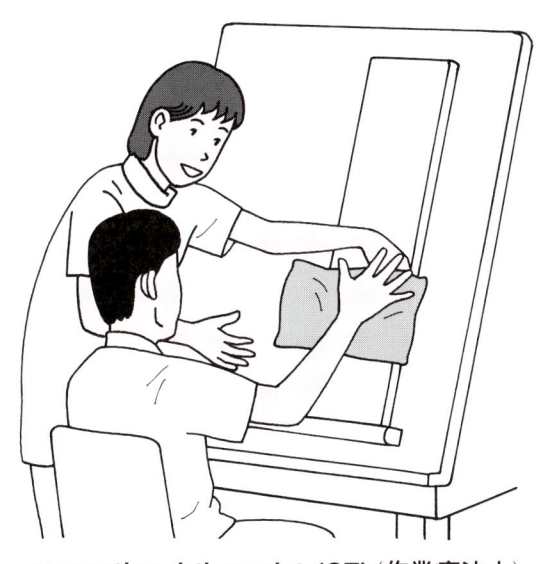

occupational therapist (OT)	作業療法士
occupational therapy	作業療法
diversional occupational therapy	気晴らし的作業療法
functional occupational therapy	機能的作業療法
supportive occupational therapy	支持的作業療法
prevocational training	職業前訓練
clay work	陶芸
leather work	革細工
metal craft	金工細工
weaving	機織り
woodworking	木工
peg board	ペグボード
sanding	サンディング(研磨)
tile mosaic	タイルモザイク

occupational therapist (OT)(作業療法士)

Chapter 13-5

(専門職種関連用語)

speech-language-hearing therapist (ST)	言語聴覚士
articulation training	構音訓練
speech and language training	言語訓練
swallowing training	嚥下訓練
eating exercise	摂食訓練
stimulation method	刺激法
writing exercise	書字訓練
auditory agnosia	聴覚失認
unilateral spatial agnosia	半側空間失認
motor aphasia	運動(性)失語
sensory aphasia	感覚(性)失語
verbal apraxia	発語失行
aspiration	誤嚥
swallowing	嚥下
prosthetist, orthotist (PO)	義肢装具士
prosthesis, limb prosthesis	義肢
upper limb prosthesis	義手
lower limb prosthesis	義足
joint	継手
orthosis, brace	装具
clinical psychologist (CP)	臨床心理士
counseling	カウンセリング
cognitive remediation	認知療法
behavior therapy	行動療法
social worker (SW)	ソーシャルワーカー
case work	ケースワーク
intake	初期面接
social welfare worker (SWW)	社会福祉士
psychiatric social worker (PSW)	精神保健福祉士

Chapter 13-5

care worker	介護福祉士
home helper	ホームヘルパー

（一般用語）

ability	能力
disablility	障害，能力障害，能力低下
disabled	肢体不自由
activities of daily living (ADL)	日常生活動作(活動)
activities parallel to daily living (APDL)	生活関連動作
activity	活動
activity limitations	活動制限
behavior	行動
development	発達
function	機能
functioning	生活機能
handicap	社会的不利
independent living (IL)	自立生活
impairment	機能障害
International Classification of Diseases and Related Health Problems (ICD)	国際疾病分類
International Classification of Functioning, Disability and Health (ICF)	国際生活機能分類
long term lying	長期臥床
participation	参加
participation restrictions	参加制約
quality of life (QOL)	生活(人生，生命)の質
rehabilitation	リハビリテーション

Chapter 13-6

Dietetics/Nutrition
(食事療法)

The dietician, nutritionist, plans what the patient should eat and when. People with diseases like diabetes, renal failure and heart disease need special diets.

Nutritionist talking to patient with high cholesterol

Health Care Professional:
　　The doctor says your cholesterol is too high.

Patient (P): Does this mean I have to lose weight?

HCP: Not really. You have to change the types of food you eat. You can eat the same amount of calories but you have to eat less fat and eat more carbohydrates.

P: I like to eat meat and dairy products.

HCP: Unfortunately, those are some of the things you will have to cut back. We also want you to eat foods that remove the bad cholesterol for your body.

P: Like what kind of food?

HCP: Fish, whole grains, certain fruits and vegetables.

P: That doesn't sound too bad.

---

nutritionist (＝dietician 栄養士)

cholesterol (コレステロール)

fat (脂肪)
carbohydrates (炭水化物)

grain (穀物)
vegetables (野菜)

Chapter 13-6

Vocabulary

nutritional condition	栄養状態
optimal nutrition	最適栄養
malnutrition	栄養障害
dietary recipe	食事箋
dietary formula	食事献立
dietary protein intake	食品蛋白摂取量
dietary fiber	食物繊維
diet	食餌(食事)
normal diet	普通食
liquid diet	流動食
semiliquid diet	半流動食
renal disease diet	腎臓病食
diabetic diet	糖尿病食
gout diet	通風病食
high fiber diet	高繊維食
low protein diet	低蛋白食
low fat diet	低脂肪食
low salt diet	低塩食
low purine diet	低プリン食
low-calorie diet	低カロリー食
salt restricted diet	塩分制限食
salt-free diet	無塩食

Other Useful Expressions

Limit intake of water, salt, potassium and phosphorus.	水分, 塩分, カリウムおよびリンの摂取を控えてください。
Restrict intake of alcohol and caffeine.	アルコールやカフェインの摂取を控えてください。

Chapter 13-7

Medication
（薬物療法）

Taking medication is an important part of treatment. Some drugs may have potent effects but also serious side effects. These drugs are available only when we have doctor's prescriptions (prescription drugs). However, we can also get some drugs having milder effects with less serious side effects, without doctor's prescription (OTC drugs).

At the pharmacy

Health Care Professional (HCP):
  Mr. (Ms) _____, please come to the counter at the pharmacy.

  pharmacy（薬局）

HCP: I'm sorry to have kept you waiting. Here are two medicines for you. One is a painkiller. I'm giving you six tablets. Take one tablet when you have pain. But don't take it unless it is necessary.

  painkiller（鎮痛薬）
  tablet（錠剤）

Patient (P): Can I take another tablet if one tablet doesn't stop the pain?

HCP: Yes, you may take at most two tablets at a time. But not over three tablets a day. Here's your antibiotic for two days. Take it four times a day, after meals and at bedtime, one capsule at a time.

  antibiotics（抗生物質）

P: What's it for?

HCP: It fights bacteria.

P: Thank you.

HCP: Take care of yourself.

Vocabulary

pharmacist	薬剤師
prescription	処方箋
over the counter (OTC)	処方箋なしに入手できる(薬)
analgesic (pain killer)	鎮痛薬(痛み止め)
anesthetic	麻酔薬
antibiotic	抗生物質
anticancer drug	抗がん薬
antidiarrhea	下痢止め
antihypertensives	降圧薬
antiphlogistic (anti-inflammatory drug)	消炎薬
antipruritic (medicine for itching)	痒み止め
antipyretic	解熱薬
antidote	解毒薬
antitussive (cough medicine)	咳止め
antiulcerative (ulcer medicine)	抗潰瘍薬
bowel medicine	整腸剤
cardiotonic	強心薬
cold medicine	風邪薬
digestive medicine	消化薬
diuretic	利尿薬

Chapter 13-7

hematinic	造血薬
laxative	緩下剤
narcoleptic (sleeping medicine)	睡眠薬
non-steroidal anti-inflammatory drug (NSAID)	非ステロイド性抗炎症薬
sedative	鎮静薬
stomach medicine	胃薬
styptic (hemostatic agent)	止血薬
tranquilizer	精神安定薬
vasopressor	昇圧薬
vitamin	ビタミン製剤
antiseptics	消毒薬
gargle, mouthwash	うがい薬
medicine for hemorrhoids	痔の薬
herbal medicine (crude extract)	生薬(漢方薬)
tablet	錠剤
capsule	カプセル
powdered medicine	散剤
granular medicine	顆粒
dry syrup	ドライシロップ
liquid medicine	液剤
sublingual medicine	舌下錠
inhalant	吸入薬
eye drops, eyewash	点眼薬
nose drops	点鼻薬
nasal spray	鼻スプレー
ointment	軟膏
eye ointment	眼軟膏
oral ointment	口腔用軟膏
suppository	坐薬
plaster	貼り薬

once a day	1日1回
twice a day	1日2回
three times a day	1日3回
four times a day	1日4回
one tablet at a time	1回1錠ずつ
when you have pain	痛いとき
when you have itching	痒いとき
when you have sleeping trouble	眠れないとき
after meals	食後に
before meals	食前に
between meals	食間に
before bedtime	就寝前に
on an empty stomach	空腹時に
with food or milk	食物またはミルクと一緒に

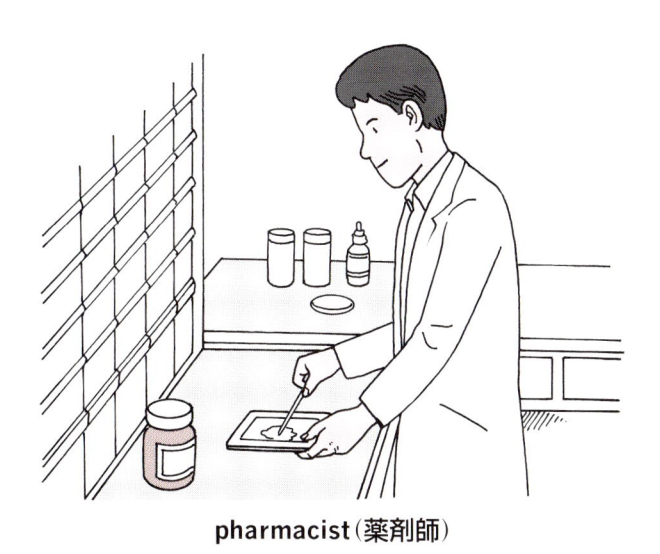

pharmacist(薬剤師)

Chapter 13-7

Other Useful Expressions

Are you allergic to any medicine? No, I'm not.	薬に対するアレルギーがありますか。いいえありません。
Take one tablet three times a day.	1日3回1錠ずつ服用してください。
Take two tablets after breakfast and after supper.	朝食後と夕食後に2錠ずつ服用してください。
Apply this cream twice a day.	このクリームを1日に2回塗ってください。
Does it have any side effects?	何か副作用がありますか。
This medicine may make you sleepy./You may feel drowsy.	眠くなることがあります。
Please don't drive a car while you're on the medicine.	この薬を服用しているときは車を運転しないでください。
Some people may have a dry cough.	空咳がでることがあります。
Keep this medicine in the refrigerator.	冷所に保存してください(冷蔵庫に保存してください)。